IT'S OK!
I HAD A STROKE

It's Ok!
I Had A Stroke

A journey of faith and healing

Sheila Lloyd

ELM HILL

A Division of
HarperCollins Christian Publishing

www.elmhillbooks.com

It's Ok! I Had A Stroke
A journey of faith and healing

Published in Nashville, Tennessee, by Elm Hill, an imprint of Thomas Nelson. Elm Hill and Thomas Nelson are registered trademarks of HarperCollins Christian Publishing, Inc.

Elm Hill titles may be purchased in bulk for educational, business, fund-raising, or sales promotional use. For information, please e-mail SpecialMarkets@ ThomasNelson.com.

Library of Congress Cataloging-in-Publication Data

Library of Congress Control Number: 2018966877

ISBN 978-1-595559616 (Paperback)
ISBN 978-1-595559425 (Hardbound)
ISBN 978-1-595559555 (eBook)

An avid journaler since my youth, I have processed feelings, circumstances, and faith through writing. When the stroke hit, I continued this practice. Therefore what you are about to read are largely my journals in real time, dated as it was happening from the night of the stroke forward. You will notice different fonts delineating our thoughts.

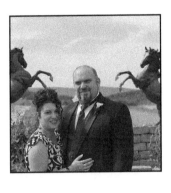

When we decided to write a book, this was the process: I would read aloud my journal entries to Brian, often on long car rides which are quite typical in Texas! Then when Brian had something to say, I would type it in. We soon found it was easier and much more enjoyable for me to simply record Brian's comments audibly and then transcribe them later, which is why you will find me occasionally inserting comments on some of Brian's reflections. I also have inserted some comments "looking back," which are printed in italics and indicated with ***.

Whether you or a loved one have suffered a stroke or you are just curious about our journey, we sincerely hope that this book will bring you encouragement and draw you closer to Jesus. We would love to hear from you! Contact us via email at sheilalloydlive2@yahoo.com Find our book and discussion page on Facebook under "IT'S OK I Had A Stroke" Or our website at www.sheilalloydlive.com.

If you are looking for help regarding stroke recovery, visit www.aBrilliantFoundation.com and contact Faith Haley 832-752-1036, outside of Katy, Texas. The custom programs she developed for Brian have brought huge steps in healing and wholeness!

Introduction

June 13, 2017

As I type this, I sit looking past a baby grand piano and stained-glass art pieces onto a desert landscape with varying shades of brown, cedar trees, and mountains in the distance. It's a landscape completely different from anything I've known my whole life, but then I suppose that is appropriate since I'm walking a journey vastly different from anything I'd ever expected. But I'm getting ahead of myself in the story. Let me back up and fill in some details.

July 9, 2014

Brian and I were high school sweethearts, best friends, married for twenty-three-and-a-half years, and have been settled in the Shenandoah Valley, Virginia (a short distance from our roots and close family ties in New Castle, Pennsylvania) nearly eighteen years. Ever since we were teenagers, we did not follow typical patterns but rather "followed the road less traveled," having pursued our dreams and ideals rather than the typical rut of jobs, careers, house in the suburbs on a cul-de-sac, etc. Brian had landed his dream job working on high-end collectible cars, restoring multimillion-dollar vehicles that won shows all over the world. I had pursued my lifelong ideal of being a stay-at-home wife and mother of two boys (Colton, nineteen at that time, and Garrett, seventeen) while teaching piano lessons in my home studio part time, composing music and recording CDs, leading worship, and serving in various ministry settings. When our younger son Garrett was born in 1997 with Down's syndrome and autism...well, that's the subject for a whole different book! Suffice it to say our lives have already been a journey where both strong faith and prayer were crucial.

Not only does Brian feel he is at the pinnacle of his career, but my studio has blossomed as well as a summer musical theater program with a friend in the area. We are enjoying our station in life probably more than ever before. The boys are gaining independence, so the family is getting a little more freedom financially, and we are situated in a home and property that we love—one we expect to remain in until death or the return of Christ, whichever comes first!

Our relationship has always been characterized by laughter, friendship, honesty, passion, music, thinking outside the box and, particularly heightened in the last several years, a deep faith in Jesus Christ that bleeds into every area of our lives.

July 10, 2014

I was up uncharacteristically before 6:00 AM, since we're in the middle of the teenage music theater camp and a very full day: camp till noon, lunch, errands, home for a few piano students, cooking dinner, hosting Bible study in the studio that evening.

Brian was up and out the door around 7:30 AM as usual heading to work—a big, burly, strong man who takes things in stride and is fairly laid back. He came home from work shortly after 5:00 PM, did some yard work and weed-whacking before dinner, held and kissed an already very weary wife, before heading out to Bible study with a couple friends in the studio across the yard.

That brings us to about 9:30 PM Thursday, July 10, 2014, when we are about to embark on the faith journey of our lives.

BRIAN'S PERSPECTIVE:

When I got up that day to go to work, I had no idea it would be the last day of my career. I came home, like Sheila said, did the normal stuff. We had to cut grass—you do that in Virginia—weed eat; I was just cleaning up because I knew people were coming over to the house for Bible study that evening. We were hosting. We had a really good discussion. People were relaxed. We were sitting out in the studio talking about God when I started noticing that something was wrong with my left arm and hand. Then I went to have a snack (still at Bible study) and I realized that I couldn't really chew right. Something was wrong.

Sheila: You felt the arm and the hand before you ate the snack?

Brian: I felt something going on; that's why I had a weird look on my face. Chuck B. is the one who noticed it. He's the one who recognized, "You're having a stroke." I didn't know what was going on at first. Did I hurt myself cutting grass or running the weed whacker? I didn't know what was going on! I just knew my left hand wouldn't work; it's like it had gone to sleep. Little did I know what faith journey God was going to take me on at that time! Sitting there with our friends laughing, joking but studying the Word of God…we wanted to learn more about God, and it's like God said, "Okay, I know this is happening. I'm going to use this to show Brian exactly Who I am."

And indeed I've learned more about God in the last couple years because I've had to cling to Him, had to rely on Him, have had to have some long hard conversations with Him. In those conversations, I'm not always in the best mood! But God always responds to me in love, peace, comfort, and in encouragement, even when I don't really think He's being fair. I complain about the Israelites as I read the Old Testament…the Hebrews wanted to go back to Egypt immediately after God had delivered them from slavery and bondage. However, God had patience with them and He has patience with me and says, "Not yet. The time is not yet." So I began to learn that quiet reliance on God which is so elusive in this world. We have so much in this world that wants to disturb our peace.

I don't know what else I can say.

Both Sheila and I feel led to share with all of you about the faith journey we were on. Our hope is just that through our being honest about what we went through—not trying to make ourselves out to be something we're not—we're just going to be open and honest and share what we felt and how God was speaking to us. Hopefully He'll use our story to encourage you or someone you know. That's our only hope. I just feel that God has taught me so much and I need to share it with others, because it involves a feeling I've been chasing my whole life. This new sense of freedom, peace, and contentment fills a life-long void in me. God has finally shown it to me out in the desert recovering from a stroke.

Sheila: Very unlikely circumstances!

Brian: Right. I thought it was going to be when I reached a certain point in my career, when we reached a certain level financially, when we retired, or when Sheila made it big in the music industry...I thought, "Well, then I'll be happy. Then I'll be content. Then I can relax and live peacefully." But I have found— God has shown me—how to live that way now. I've learned how to live peacefully and contentedly without any of that stuff. And you, too, can learn it! God wants to teach those lessons to everyone. But you're not going to learn them just by listening to me. You're going to learn them by listening to Him and what He has to say. He wrote us a book that has those truths in it. We just need to believe what He has to say.

We invite you to come with us on this journey if you dare, and we'll share with you what God has taught us. If you let Him, He can teach you the same thing.

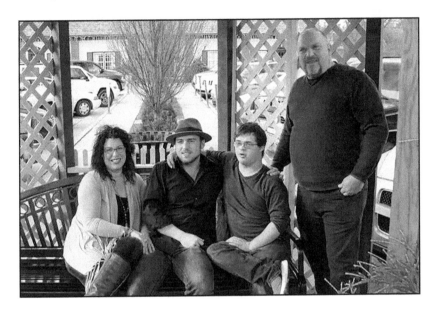

THE NIGHT OF THE STROKE

Sheila: What I remember from the earliest moments of the stroke:

We had finished Bible study and prayer time, followed by my playing "Turn Your Eyes Upon Jesus" on the piano. I asked Brian if he was going to play guitar with me and he said, "No, not this time. You play." Little did I know that would be the last time he could've played with me for many months.

At the close of the prayer, Brian started talking emphatically, passionately, about insights he'd received from the story of Job in the Bible (which was **not** the topic we'd been studying that evening) … "It's all about surrender, it's **all** about **God**! Not us." Brian was making statements along the lines of, "Jesus is everything to me. God is number one in my life. Not my wife, not my job, not my kids, not my cars or talents. It's all about Jesus! I don't care what Satan ever wants to throw at me, I will praise Jesus!" He had tears in his eyes as he said it, and I was so touched by his firm statement of commitment (although admittedly I gulped a bit at that kind of challenge thrown into the spiritual air!) I had heard him say similar things several times over the last year or two, but this was such a strong, decisive statement.

Right after his statement, I passed him a tray of appetizers our friends had brought. It was chunks of summer sausage, cheese, and pineapple on a toothpick. Brian took one and slid all three bites into his mouth off the toothpick all at once. I looked at him a couple seconds later, and he had a strange look on his face. It looked as though he didn't want to chew it. I thought, "Oh that's right, he doesn't like pineapple." So I said to him, "Just spit out the pineapple if you don't like it." He was shaking his head kind of oddly, and it seemed as though the food was getting bigger in his cheeks instead of smaller, as it should have if he had chewed and swallowed. You know, in those circumstances you don't want to stare at someone. But when I glanced over a moment later and he still was struggling, I couldn't figure out what was wrong.

Then our friend asked him, "Brian, can you stand up?" Brian rolled his head from side to side oddly. Our friend asked, "Can you raise your left arm?" Brian reached over with his right hand, grabbed his left wrist, raised his left arm above his head, and then let go. His left arm fell down and hit him in the head. At that point I noticed his left cheek was sagging slightly. And he was sweating all over. We all immediately gathered around him and prayed for him.

I thought to myself, "Maybe he's allergic to pineapple. He's having a weird allergic reaction. We'll get him to the hospital, get him some meds to counteract the allergic reaction and be on our way. After all, I have a musical camp production tomorrow morning!" I'm really not sure I would've even known what a stroke was at that point.

I ran to the house, got a towel and an ice pack, and came back. Our friends were still gathered around him praying and trying to help him. I asked one of them, "What should I do?" She said emphatically, "Call 911 now!" I did.

I have to say the overwhelming sense in the room was the peace that passes all understanding, the incredible peace and presence of the Holy Spirit. Our studio had been bathed in worship, prayer, and Bible study not only that evening but for years. Therefore, fear was honestly not the primary emotion in either Brian or me that night. That alone is a miracle! One only explained by the grace and presence of the Lord Jesus.

The ambulance arrived within 15 minutes, came in and very expertly evaluated him, transferred him on a stretcher, and loaded him in the back of the ambulance. After grabbing my purse and having my friends' assurance that they would stay with the kids, I got in the front seat of the ambulance.

At that point the surreal realization of what was happening began to dawn on me. Brian passed me his I AM SECOND bracelet that he had worn for quite some time. I cried realizing that was where his mind was. The team was working on him in the back of the ambulance. We drove up Interstate 81 North at—I'm not sure how many —miles per hour. I quickly called my mother to pray and put a shout out on Facebook, "We need prayers right now!" I think I also texted Bryan and Aimee Patrick (pastor and wife at our church, Fresh Water Fellowship, which we had helped them start in 2012; also some of our very best friends). They were on vacation in Georgia. I said something to the driver who was very quiet. I said I was praying. She said, "I am too!" I didn't say anything else, letting her concentrate on driving and praying.

I remember staring at the road praying, knowing the Lord was with me but also realizing, "I could be a widow tonight and be raising two teenage boys by myself."

Some friends met us in the emergency room in Winchester Medical Center, and Brian was whisked back for evaluation. His parents arrived soon after, and by this time I obviously was deeply concerned. It was definitely not any kind of allergic reaction, and it appeared that the situation was incredibly serious, even life-threatening. We hugged each other and cried, prayed, and waited. Brian was taken for more than one CT scan, and they told me he was getting sick, vomiting. (Vomiting is a very bad thing, especially when you are having bleeding on the brain!)

Finally, I think it was around midnight, doctors informed me they did believe it was a brain bleed stroke. They wanted him to have the best possible care, but they did not have a neurologist on staff at that facility. They were asking my permission to fly him by helicopter to INOVA Fairfax. Of course I gave permission. This entire time Brian was conscious and aware of what was happening, responsive when I or anyone spoke to him. He seemed mentally cognizant, alert, and very much at peace although his speech was extremely slow and slurred.

Brian was prepared for the helicopter ride, while his parents and I drove the two-plus hours to Fairfax, Virginia. When we arrived, it was after 2:00 AM. We sat down in the waiting room and a staff member said the helicopter had just landed. Then one of the attendants handed me Brian's wedding ring. They said it was better for him not to have a ring on that hand for now. That's when I really broke down, staring at his wedding ring in my hand.

The nurse informed me they had installed a breathing tube while he was on the helicopter. But she made a point of emphasizing they asked his permission to do it. He gave permission to do it. I realized later the significance of this was that he was conscious, coherent, and able to make that decision. That is very rare in a stroke! Usually the patient is unconscious and unresponsive. They also emphasized he did not receive the breathing tube because he was having trouble breathing. They put the breathing tube in so that he would receive meds and go to sleep, which would stop the vomiting. As I said, when your brain is bleeding, you do not want to have the violent reaction of vomiting added to the mix.

I would often walk into the bathroom just to collect my thoughts and pray. What I wanted to say was, "Lord, please stop this right now! Just make him fine again!" However, it was as though the Holy Spirit would not let those words come out of my mouth. Instead, what I felt led to pray repeatedly was, "Oh Lord God, please do not let this last one minute longer than absolutely necessary in order to accomplish everything You want to accomplish. And also please Lord, have mercy on us."

After a few moments I would leave the bathroom and enter the surreal, overstimulating world of ER. I would stand or sit by my husband's side, not understanding what was going on and how he was going to be OK again. His blood pressure was very high, and his color slightly grayish green. But again, he was responsive to questioning and able to give intelligent albeit very slurred appropriate answers. They kept asking him, "Do you know what day it is? Do you know what the date is? Do you know what the year is? Do you know the president's name?" After this series of questions several times, Brian made a joke. At that point the techs laughed and said, "He's going to be OK."

They were having a very difficult time getting his blood pressure stabilized. I think one of the highest readings was 195/105. I remember a small curtained-off room, very kind doctors and nurses but with somber, serious, focused expressions on their faces. They were not saying very much, just trying to get him stabilized. Brian's parents and I tried to stay out of the way, but there was no way we were leaving his side. They finally transferred him up to ICU, as there was a whole stroke unit in that hospital. By then I think it was about 4:30 AM. I realized I have been up and in full gear for almost 24 hours. I often have trouble with my sugar dropping if I'm overtired or haven't eaten enough. I had no headache whatsoever and felt fine. I'm sure some of that was the adrenaline! One of the nurses did give me an Ensure drink, which I appreciated. Although I was extremely concerned, I felt the Lord's presence and hand on me.

I remember the doctor when Brian finally got settled in ICU. It was about 4:30 AM. The doctor was rather young and had a look of grave concern on his face when he turned to me in response to my question, "He's going to be all right now, isn't he?" I could tell he was trying to be encouraging and yet honest as he said, "This is going to be a long process. It's a marathon not a sprint. But for right now, Brian is stable and resting. The next 24 hours will tell us quite a bit."

That was an extremely sobering statement to hear! But I needed it to brace myself for the journey ahead and hold on tightly to the Lord! I also realized that I needed rest. So as difficult as it was to leave my husband's side, I convinced my mother-in-law to get a hotel room and a few hours of sleep. Brian's dad refused to leave and spent the night (what was left of it since hospitals spring to life at the crack of dawn!) on the chair beside his son.

Waking up in the hotel room a few hours later July 11, 2014 was one of the lowest points of my life. Dressed in the same clothes for 24 hours, far from home, my children, my dog, and my toothbrush! Reality throws gaunt, boney fingers of pain, despair and threatens fear… and a crack laces its way across the glass windshield of your life. Where am I? What's going on? Oh God, no! You mean this is actually real? There's no way to go back to sleep. Check the cell phone for streams of texts and voicemails coming in… friends and family shocked, praying. Talked voice to voice with a couple people. Cried harder than I had yet in this ordeal. Held my mother-in-law, comforting each other in this foreign, opaque reality. Opened the curtain letting daylight of a midsummer morning into the room. How could the sun still be shining like usual? Hate to think of something as mundane as my stomach, but I'm starving. Pull ourselves together and face the day. We head back to ICU. Surreal. "You promise to lead the blind, Lord." Okay.

Brian:

As I started to understand what was happening, I realized I was losing function although I had no pain at all. You know, when you're suddenly unable to move…. When the squad arrives, that's a sobering feeling… when you can't even put yourself on the stretcher. These strangers have to pick you up, move you, and put you on the stretcher. You see your wife trying to be strong, but you see the worry and despair in her eyes. I didn't even get to see my kids. Just heard friends say they would stay with the kids. Then you're watching the house—all you hold dear in the world, really—disappear through the back window of the ambulance as it pulls out the driveway. I realized I might be facing the end of all I was and would be in the world.

You never know how you'll react to that until you're faced with such a situation—that's where the rubber meets the road. You're faced with the fact that this could very well be the end of your life as you know it. Either you're okay with that or you're not.

I surrendered everything I was at that point and said, "Jesus, if this is my time then that's fine. Take me home with You. If you have something left for me to do here, then fine. I'll be glad to stay with my wife and kids." At that point, I felt this incredible sense of peace wash over me. It wasn't like I knew how things were going to turn out—flying down the highway in an ambulance and people working on you—but I knew that either way it was okay. It seemed like the spiritual battle had not been decided one way or another yet—almost like my life hung in the balance of the shift of power. But either way my soul was secure.

When I was in the ER things really got exciting—all these doctors working on me. I got sick (vomiting), couldn't talk, needed a tube in me to help me from getting sick, was rushed back and forth for CAT scans, MRIs, etc. Then there was a point—maybe when they put me on the helicopter or maybe before—but at some point I felt my body relax. I heard the Spirit of God say, "You're going to be okay, because I'm not done with what I want you to do yet." Not like it was that I had to grow more. It was as if God said, "There's more you have to do. It's going to be hard and it's going to be long, but you're going to teach other people in the process." I felt this incredible peace, and I wasn't worried about it anymore. The next thing I knew, I woke up in ICU. I was never scared. Never angry. Frustrated later, yes, because you can't do what you want—that's the flesh—but I was never scared or angry at that point.

Now looking back from today (over two years later)...I realize it was about truly surrendering everything. We say we do when we repent...and we do. But at that point it was a complete relinquishment of everything I was. For most people at the point of salvation, we are not faced with life or death physically. God showed me through this experience that thank God, I was able to surrender **everything**... *"Okay, either take me or use me. You're God; I'm not. I'm simply yours." At that point God becomes very, very real to you!*

Sheila's journal notes reflecting on the night of stroke: these are scattered notes because that is the way one's mind often works in crisis.

Very clear it's a test... lots of fours (number of testing). Several times I noticed clock at 4:44... AM and PM. Mom and my hotel room at 5:30 AM Friday was 114. He is in the 7 South tower ICU Room 715. Seven is the Biblical number of perfection and completion.

"Be still and know that I am God." Psalm 46:10 NIV

Exodus 14:14 (NIV) word from the Lord to me in the ambulance: "The Lord will fight for you; you need only to be still."

"And they overcame him [Satan] by the blood of the Lamb and by the word of their testimony!" Revelation 12:11(KJV)

Pray that Brian's bodily systems will stabilize in Jesus' name. Command wholeness and strength to return and bind any retaliatory spirits in the name of Jesus.

Grizzly bear...

And how M (a prayer warrior) saw it retreat into the woods... victory is at hand, major breakthrough coming. That was minutes before the doctor came out with the good investigative procedure report.

NO FEAR allowed entrance!

Later, M said that in her vision the gate had been left open. That's how the grizzly bear was allowed into the yard. She said she didn't know for sure but had the sense that gate was "taking care of your health." I got the same message from the Lord before she said it. God had been warning Brian for months to change his eating and exercise habits because God had assignments for him. I had to repent as well, because I knew he wasn't taking some of his meds. Forgive us, Lord, and I ask for your mercy.

Perspiring... detoxing his body in all realms

"No weapon formed against you will prosper." Isaiah 54:17 (NKJV)

Romans 8:26–28 (NIV) "In the same way, the Spirit helps us in our weakness. We do not know what we ought to pray for, but the Spirit himself intercedes for us through wordless groans. And he who searches our hearts knows the mind of the Spirit, because the Spirit intercedes for God's people in accordance with the will of God. And we know that in all things God works for the good of those who love him, who have been called according to his purpose."

A friend, while praying for us, was led to Psalm 28 for me and Psalm 39 for Brian.

Psalm 68:35 (NIV) "You, God, are awesome in your sanctuary; the God of Israel gives power and strength to his people. Praise be to God!"

1 John 2:14 (NIV) "I write to you, dear children, because you know the Father. I write to you, fathers, because you know him who is from the beginning. I write to you, young men, because you are strong, and the word of God lives in you, and you have overcome the evil one."

Encouraging word from a friend out of state via email:
"If you are committed to the fire, you can't negotiate the flames!"
Quote by Arthur Burt. Yep, Lord, I needed to hear that right now. Thanks!

Proverbs 3:5–6 (NIV): "Trust in the Lord with all your heart and lean not on your own understanding; in all your ways submit to him, and he will make your paths straight."

First Few Days

These are entries from the Facebook Group page, which is the main way I kept people updated throughout this process:

From Sheila July 11 or 12, 2014:
Brian had a brain bleed stroke and mild heart attack Thursday night. We are at INOVA Fairfax ICU. He is making great progress, and we are seeing the Lord's hand. We fully stand on Jesus' healing and know that he will have total recovery in God's perfect timing. Process goes ICU, step-down unit, and then rehab facility, although we also know God can do a spontaneous miracle! Pray for strength and movement to return to his left side and clearer speech and writing... COMPLETE wholeness and restoration in Jesus' name. Thank you so much for caring and praying and whatever the Lord lays on your heart to do to help, we humbly accept and greatly appreciate!

From the friend who created the group:
Ways to contribute to immediate financial needs.... As you know, the biggest blessings to Brian and Sheila Lloyd are your fervent prayers and praises to the Lord—AND there are current real financial needs. Anything at all helps. At this point it is not known how long Brian will be in the hospital, so Sheila and Brian's parents are traveling back and forth daily, tag-teaming with staying overnight. They need $ for extended-stay

lodging, meals, and gas. The hotel cost alone is around $750 for 8 nights. Not having to worry about funds would be a huge comfort as Brian recovers. Money may be contributed by mailing checks made out to Fresh Water Fellowship, Woodstock VA. For more immediate service, call Aimee Patrick.

*** *Taking assessment of Brian's current situation: Written in 2017, looking back....*

As far as the severity of the brain bleed stroke: Brian lost absolutely all movement on his entire left side. I remember him lying in bed in the ER as well as ICU and even at the beginning of rehab. They would say, "Brian, can you wiggle your left big toe?" I would look at his left foot expectantly—so would he— but there would be nothing, no movement. He could feel if they pricked him with a needle or touched him. But he could not move his left foot at all. Same with his hand and arm. He could move his shoulder slightly, which they found promising and interesting. The drooping of the face did not seem to last too long. However, the double vision lasted for a few weeks.

Even his right side was weakened in many ways, still is, even after three years out. While he was still in ICU, I had taken a short break to eat or something. When I came back to his room, I noticed an 8 1/2 x 11 piece of paper on the bulletin board with "Brian Lloyd" written in longhand with a marker. It looked like maybe a four-year-old had written it, slanted and sprawled across the paper. In fact, a therapist had been there. Brian had written that himself—with his RIGHT hand. That was extremely difficult for me to digest! I quickly recovered and was celebratory and encouraging; but I remember that being a moment I truly wondered what the future would hold.

Because even his mouth, tongue, and swallowing was affected, he was on a liquid diet at first and then a very soft diet for several weeks. I remember this packet of thickener we'd have to put in even his water to drink. It was kind of nasty, and he really didn't like it! We tried putting it in Ginger Ale ... didn't help much. Certainly not in coffee! He was so excited the day he didn't have to use that thickener stuff anymore! But that was several weeks later. I think when he came home from rehab—five weeks after the stroke—there were still some things we were supposed to thicken for him. This of course helped avoid choking.

His work with the speech therapist involved many different aspects— from cognition, pronunciation, to even tongue exercises and stimulation of the inside of the mouth.

The first time a PT visited him in ICU, he brought along an assistant. I watched these two men kindly, with great patience and encouragement, help my 285-pound husband sit on the side of the bed. He was like dead weight, could barely balance himself even sitting. And of course he was very tired with the effort! They did eventually get him to transfer to a chair—which involved precarious seconds in between. One of the therapist was a rather small man, and Brian was joking and concerned that he would fall and crush him. Brian's sense of humor and graciousness to others through the whole thing was amazing to watch.

Therapy in the residential rehab was intense! He had visits from physical therapy while in INOVA Fairfax, VA, but residential rehab was a whole different story. It was a blessing that he was even able to go. They couldn't transfer him until his heart and blood pressure were stable enough to endure the 3–4-hour per day of various therapies. A couple weeks into the process since he showed true motivation, a great attitude as well as physical and mental improvement, the therapists would work with him as much as he could handle, putting in extra time to help him.

BRIAN: I can't say enough about therapists in the residential rehab and later in outpatient rehab. They're so patient, kind, helpful, and truly have your best interest at heart. They work their hardest to get you back to proper functioning. I saw so many people (other patients) get angry. True, there were times it was frustrating—for them and for me—I wanted so badly to do something but couldn't. But the therapists were always patient, encouraging, and uplifting.

Sheila: I remember when he got home he couldn't even open a water bottle for himself. He could not grip it hard enough in his left hand to allow his right hand to open it; and he did not have the fine motor strength in his left hand to open it while his right hand gripped it. Realizing that was a very difficult thing for both of us. For a few weeks I had to help put his socks on, tie his shoes, and anything else he needed. He had to wear pants only with elastic waist bands for quite a while because he was not able to do the buttons. There were so many things that came so easily before—millions of movements we make every hour that we don't even think about. Now his body just wouldn't cooperate.

However, we learned later that the type of stroke he had—a sub arachnoid hematoma on the right side, at the base of the brainstem— very often leaves victims paralyzed physically, extremely compromised mentally if not dead. So we were thankful! And once again we saw the hand of God.

BRIAN: REFLECTION ON JULY 11, 2014

When I woke up in ICU and realized the full extent of what had happened…I can't move, I'm bedridden…your mind goes all over the place. I guess you desperately search to find "normal" because normal is gone. You don't go to work, you don't cut the grass. You're stuck in a bed with tubes in you and nurses have to help you do everything. Suddenly you only have your right side of your body to help you do anything, and even that was sketchy. I can't even watch TV because my brain is too confused and it gives me a headache.

When you're left lying in bed for hours and hours at a time thinking, your mind can go all sorts of places. God protected me. The battle had been fought and over by that time. Now it was a time of God protecting me from myself. My own mind didn't go into depression and despair. A big part of that protection was that Sheila and my parents were right there. My wife was a pillar of strength. This experience showed me how strong my wife was in the Lord because she clung to Him. I did too because that's all I had! I told God, "You've let everything be taken away and now You will give it back to me in the order You want, in the way You desire and in the proper perspective." Cars were gone. My work on Ferraris—gone. Being the big strong person in the room was gone. The music was gone.

My life was cars, music, and being the big strong guy in the room. In any situation, I could always either fix it, pick it up, or play it. If I couldn't fix it, I could at least move it. Now all that was gone and I had to rely on God to fix things, move things, and make things work.

Yes, I was able to let go. He gave me grace to do it, but it was still hard because I had to change my mindset. The answer was not for me to try to figure out a way to do it. I couldn't because my brain was still rebooting. Yes I could talk (extremely slurred for a few days though) and joke—I still had sense of humor—but my thoughts were still a little jumbled.

God put people in my life who really stepped up...my boss and his wife, guys I worked with, church family, Bryan and Aimee Patrick...and I have to say just a little bit about them right here: we really saw what true friends they were. As busy as their lives were, they really made time to minister extremely to both of us. It made me appreciate them on a whole new level, and they will always be very dear friends. Aimee was willing to just drop everything to be at a friend's side to help meet a need without expecting anything in return. Laying her life down like Christ said. Bryan too—he worked so many hours and then pastored a church, but he made the effort to come and minister to me. It was really special. You will hear their names often in this book because truly, they stood right beside us the whole time.

During that time, it was like I switched off one part of my brain and switched on another. God said, "Look, this stinks, and you're going to have to deal with this for a period of time. Realize you can't do this stuff. Don't even try. Just let Me do it." And He did! God parted the waters! Yes Sheila was behind the scenes and also Aimee, working hard at all the administrative details. But God did it. And before the stroke I would have felt bad that someone was doing so much for me...but God gave me grace to accept the help. I had to accept it. In my weakness He is strong. It's time in my life to let Him do things! Quit trying to do them on my own. God reminded me, "Physically you can't do anything. Just concentrate on the therapy."

July 12??, 2014

Good progress every day! Trying to speak more and able to feed himself with his right hand (strictly a soft diet to avoid choking). Pray specifically that BP will remain low and stable, so he can get off IV meds and be transferred out of ICU. Also pray double vision goes away and of course all strength to return quickly to his left side through the name and power of Jesus! Thanks.

Tonight was such a blessing...well, overall it was a good day with increased speech, seeing his personality and his sense of humor. He and I had some private time, so were able to have some heart-to-heart talks, which was a blessing. Bryan and Aimee visited tonight, and he was laughing and making wise cracks (speech still slurred)...did my heart **such** good! Praise God!

PLEASE pray that his BP stabilizes and remains low so he can get rid of the IV BP meds. Until he gets rid of that drip he cannot leave ICU. They have tried lowering the dosage and his BP shoots up.

So BP, full motion on left side, and clear vision are the immediate needs. No, we have no idea yet how long he'll be in the hospital. Thanks!

*** *Looking back, I remember at this time having such a mix of emotions. I am the "Type A" personality who gets calm during a crisis. I seem to keep a clear head and just do what needs to be done. Certainly I had times of emotional breakdown, when the reality of the situation* *would overwhelm me and I would desperately just want things to go back to normal. Early on in this process I just was focused on Brian getting better. I wanted to be right by his side and to do whatever I could to help him. It was such a strange feeling to see my big, bold, strong-as-an-ox, football-player build husband in such a weak and vulnerable position. But truly, from the first moments, I had a peace from the Lord and a firm sense in my spirit that he was going to eventually be restored. In the meantime, I was just focusing on day by day—doing what needed to be done and trying to see positive steps.*

BRIAN REFLECTING ON FLIPPING THE WORK SWITCH… recorded on 8/9/17 after hearing a close friend was in ICU with ministroke and extremely high BP.

Talking about men at our age (late forties) and the things that weigh heavily on their minds…your career, dealing with questions such as "Am I measuring up with the success of others?" "Am I a good provider?" Then as your kids get older, you wonder if you've raised them to be successful. All these things that the world tells you you've got to do—like the Law of Moses—you've got to check all these boxes. So you worry, "Did I handle this right?"

Sheila: There's no way we can.

Brian: No one gets it all right. So then your kids are in their early twenties or you're getting towards fifty and you realize, "The greater part of my life is over. It's too late to do much about it now. My gosh, I've failed." In a lot of ways it feels like that. However, Christ is there to say, "No! You didn't! You're not a failure." If we turn to Christ or rely on Christ we hear that, but so many people refuse to turn to Him. If we choose to stay in the common culture's philosophy, we don't realize that. Even if we are saved—we are actually Christians, but we're still adhering to the world's mentality trying to measure up to a level of what the world says is successful or what is acceptable. None of us can measure up! Very few people ever can—at least some people *appear* as though they are attaining that level. From the outside looking in, they look like they have measured up and are successful by the world's standards.

We see them and think, "Man! Why can't I be like that? Gosh dang it, I did x again. I was this way or that way. I let this go. I let this slip by. I did this or didn't do this...." That pressure builds up! Over time with those thoughts, fears, and worries piling on, at some point it blows off—whether it's a stroke, a heart attack, or maybe some other kind of trauma or health issue. That's why a lot of people around this age get divorced—people just want to hit the "reset" button, but you can't.

Without Christ, you cannot reset things. With Christ, that pressure is gone because there is no "having to measure up" to any kind of level of achievement. It's just simply the mentality of "I love Jesus. I'm His." That's what God requires of me. That's what He wants from me.

So I understand completely what is going through people's minds at this point in life. I'm sure it's not just men. I'm sure women feel those things too.

Sheila: Talk a little bit about the "provider" aspect. You said you realized that as soon as you were in the ambulance.

Brian: I was so geared to working to provide for my family—so you could stay home, take care of the kids, and give piano lessons.

Sheila: I was the more nurturing one.

Brian: Yes. And you handled the household so well. I was trained from the time I was little that the man goes to work. We work hard. We work a lot of hours. We don't take off just because the wind is blowing the wrong way. You go to work when you're sick. You go to work when you'd rather not or when things aren't right. You go to work in bad weather. You work! Once in a while I took off for doctor's appointments or things like that.

Sheila: But you didn't like it! You'd get angry at me for scheduling them!

Brian: No, I didn't like it. I would fuss. So you work. But when something happens, like the stroke that is out of your control, your perspective changes very quickly. I couldn't control it, and I knew it right away.

Sheila: Well, you couldn't move!

Brian: Yeah. In my mind I went through the various scenarios very quickly…if I don't make it through this, she'll have the life insurance policy. She'll be okay.

Sheila: In some ways that's like you still provided.

Brian: Yes, it's like, "I'm good on that one because I had that taken care of." But if I live through it, then what?? I knew at the very least I wasn't going to be able to work for a while. How are we going to survive? Your mind goes through all that. Fortunately, the Lord had already been intensely at work in my life for a couple years. I had been reading the Bible avidly. I was able to think and say, "Wait. I know that the promises in God's word say that I am in His hands. He is the Provider, not me. He provides for my family, not me. He may provide by giving me a job to do but it's His provision, not mine. He will continue to provide even if He chooses to let me go through something where I can't work." So I had to just lay it down, give it all to Him and say, "Here, Jesus, You take care of this because I can't anymore. At least not for a while. I can't. You're going to have to do it." And He promises that He will! He'd been doing it the whole time anyway. I just didn't realize it. That's a hard thing for a man. It's humbling. You want to fight, kick, scream, and hold on to the life you've created—the life the world says matters. You want to hold on to that bondage that you've let yourself get into because that's all you know.

Sheila: Wasn't it hard for you when you realized you couldn't work?

Brian: Not that much. Because if you're in that situation, by then you've already turned the switch off in your head. By the time I woke up and realized that I survived, then within 12 hours or so I figured, "I'm retired."

Sheila: Really? I mean, I remember your making the comment soon after you woke up saying, "I think the Ferrari gig is up," but I didn't realize you had already settled that in your mind. I would think that'd be really hard for a man because of your identity being wrapped up in what you did and also because of the whole provider thing.

Brian: Well, you go through various scenarios in your head, and you go through them fast! I mean, it only takes minutes to work through these thoughts. So in my mind I woke up and thought, "I'm done. I had a good run, and I enjoyed what I did. I might do it again part time. Hopefully I'll get strong enough to enjoy it … but I'm done doing it the way I always have." And I was fine with that. Now there are days when you get frustrated because you want to try to do something but you can't do it. That's a different deal. That's the situation—not the long-term, the big picture. The big picture is that I knew when I woke up that my life had forever changed, whatever that meant. It was going to look very different from here on out.

If you are reading this and are in a similar situation, I would say this to you: it might sound weird, but give it all to God. He will take care of it. He will prove Himself to be faithful. Your life may or may not change on the outside, but take this time to let it change on the inside. Get to know Jesus better. Read the Bible. I can't emphasize that enough. That has changed my life so much these last three years. My attitude is just different. What else can I say? Let Jesus show you how different it's going to be.

July 15, 2014

Photo of my right hand … racing stripe band gets me in to see Brian 24/7. His I AM SECOND bracelet he handed to me during the initial ambulance ride Thursday night. He wanted to let me know where his mind was … "It's ALL about God!" I

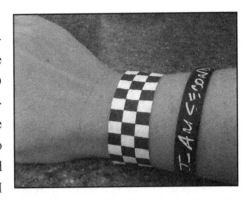

asked him yesterday if he wanted it back yet. He shook his head. So I will wear it until I give it back to him. Great reminder! You can google "I am second" or look on YouTube and hear testimonies.

Just got a call from Brian's mom, Wanda Lloyd, as I am home today, and his folks are at hospital. Huge praise! Therapists had Brian sitting on edge of bed with legs swung over side. He was able to push with his left leg **and** his left arm! Also, when the nurse was lifting his left arm she could feel his muscle helping her. They were so thrilled! They have decreased the IV BP med slightly and his pressure is still good, so they will try to decrease it again. Goal is to move him **out** of ICU today! Go God!

Keep praying and expect more miracles.

Wanda just texted. They have stopped the IV BP med drip and feel they may have the right combination! Of course they do! We have been praying for God's perfect number for his blood pressure. He hears and answers prayer. Praise you Lord!

July 16, 2014

Wonderful time in personal worship in the studio this morning. God gave me a song through 1Chronicles 29:11–13 ... worship IS warfare! Music has always been a powerful way for me to process emotions as well as to draw close to the Lord in any kind of circumstance. So I was really thankful to have that opportunity today!

Just talked to his nurse in ICU. She is his favorite at this point because she brought him orange sherbet. Not to be outdone, his night nurse brought him two Sunday night. Brian has informed the first that she has competition! His sense of humor is intact.

Anyway, he has been off the IV drip since she left yesterday (probably about 7:30 PM). They haven't written the orders for transfer yet, as doctors want to make sure his BP is stable.

So continue to pray! Looking forward to visit from Rob and Tammy Wescoat today! Rob is a barber and is going to get him all spiffed up. I can finally have a say in how long his goatee is. Lol.

He has been cleared to be transferred out of ICU ... waiting for an available bed.

Heart doctor said ... they will do a stress test tomorrow morning just to make sure his heart is ready for "acute rehab" ... This means he will be going to a facility where they'll work him three hours/day. It's great because it shows that they believe he is strong enough and showing great progress to warrant that.

OT had him moving hips back and forth in bed. He was able to push some with his left arm and leg. With help they had him standing, getting up and down, sitting (few seconds without support), and then moved over to a chair! All great work! Praise God!

I asked him how he felt when we were alone and he was in the chair. He said, "This is hard." (Meaning the physical work involved.) But he also knows and believes that the Lord will totally restore him. Timing is in God's hands.

Perhaps what made him the most excited was when the Occupational Therapist put tape on a pair of (nonprescription) eyeglasses which removed the double vision. He said, "That is amazing! How did you do that?"

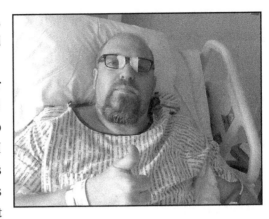

Thank you all for your love, prayers, and support! We feel it. Please keep praying for miracles…I am asking God for his mercy to keep this test as short as possible but that it will still accomplish his perfect will.

Brian: talking about nurses, therapists, and staff

The first week in ICU and step down unit at INOVA, Fairfax, VA showed me how hard these people work to take care of you! They have such compassion. Although they have hard jobs, they get little appreciation from their patients. So much of time people are in pain or unconscious. They don't get many thank-yous. I was conscious the whole time, but they still did a lot for me because I couldn't. They do so, so much! They care for you.

I remember one of my ICU nurses expressing his faith (not Christianity) to his friend in the hall. He was a really good nurse who showed me much compassion. Although I couldn't communicate with him, I wondered—how much more compassion would he have if he knew Christ? Everyone did a really thorough job: it was obvious they were well trained. I wondered, do they have compassion or are they doing it for a paycheck? I think they had some compassion. But as a Christian you realize that compassion will not save them. Human compassion is coming from the flesh…their desire to be a good person or fulfill a career. It's not focused on Christ. And if it's not focused on Christ, then it's all for naught. The thing that matters is our relationship with Jesus. When we have that secure, He directs our path. His grace, his compassion, his mercy are shown through us to others. That's true compassion, true grace, true mercy.

As friends, family, and work associates came in to see me, I could see that they were trying to be positive— to put on good face; but I could see behind their eyes there was just sadness and fear. Some of it was fear for me, but some of it was because it reminded them of their mortality. What God started to drive home to me at that point (and continued through this whole process) is that this life is just a tiny speck of the reality of life in God. Why do we cling to this life when we have the promise and hope of eternity through Jesus? But people think this world, this existence, is all we have... we try to hold it, protect it, and cling to it. Just give it up! Give it to God.

At that point I began to let go... yes, in the first moments of the stroke, I started to give up and surrender, but really in ICU is where the process crystalized. I realized I'm not me anymore. I was reminded of the song I wrote, "Take Me, Change Me Lord"... take me, use me... Jesus, make me more like You.

At that point I started to understand that God is using this—He let Satan tear me down so that HE could build me back up. God didn't cause the stroke, but He allowed it. Looking back now I see that God knew I was not really going to be able to give up my life. I loved my life—I thought God had really let me find a type of nirvana. I had found this little place to work where I could hone my craft and almost hide away. Even local people don't really even know it's there. I could just go two miles to work and come back. I felt like I had found a little niche, and I could just wait out life—we could just have a nice quiet little existence, just be there for the rest of our lives.

But God was wanting us to do something different.

We had felt the pull to Texas as an adventure of faith. I felt the pull, but I couldn't let go of what I had because it was just so much of me, who I was, what my flesh totally wanted. God wanted to show me that's not who I am. Who I am is in Jesus, not defined by what I do. He let Satan strip away what I thought defined me, so that He could build me back up in who I really am in Jesus. On the night of stroke I realized. "Well, God didn't take me."

We go through life and we try to control things. Then this stroke comes and takes away all control. You're left with just you and God. You realize God is just God. He's the same as He always was.

Things were really going well for us...we were happy. Financially things seemed like they were finally working. We thought we were okay, had a lot of friends, playing a lot of music, doing a lot of stuff. We thought we were doing something significant, things were finally clicking. Later, I realized I was trying to do it.

There was an awakening in me, but I couldn't let go of my life in the flesh—my house, my career, my music, my cars. I had wrapped up my identity thinking that's how God made me. God wanted to break it down into the simple truth: without God I'm nothing. With Christ, I'm everything.

I'm not saying everyone who wants to get close to Christ has to go through a trauma! God will bring all of us to a point in our lives when we come to the end of ourselves. Hopefully for you, it won't be that drastic!

I thought I was strong. My philosophy often was, "I'm going to make things fit." For a lot of my life, by force of will I got things done my way. I just kept going forward by my own strength and shaped my life into what I thought was right. God brought me to the end of myself and me: "No longer can you look the world in the eye and say, 'Come here, I'll take you on!' God showed me that in my weakness I am the strongest in Him.

He has me. I know that I'm with him forever. I felt that in the ambulance. There was no sense of dread trying to hang on to my life. Just let the people do the work and whatever happens is fine. He showed me that at the end of my strength, there He is! I was "saved" since I accepted Jesus at eleven years old as my Savior.

But until that night I'm not really sure if I had ever made Him Lord of my life.

July 14, 2014
The wonder glasses.

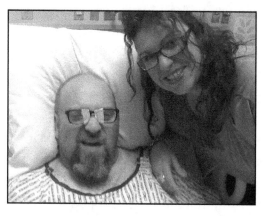

Well, he has his new room... still south tower, floor 3, room 364, bed 1. Gotta say I know it is **such** a blessing that he is strong enough to be out of ICU, but they certainly spoil you with the accommodations up there! We are now in a little tiny room but that's okay! Hopefully he will soon be transferred to an "acute rehab facility" in the next day or so.

His roommate's name is William. From the other side of the curtain he heard me say that we were worship leaders and musicians, and he clapped his hands! Turns out he is too, as well as a pianist, singer/song-writer. How cool, huh? He talked to me for quite a while about what the Lord Jesus has done for him ... among other things, carrying him through a stroke, heart attack, seizures... So we'll probably have a worship service in there soon. Pray for us as we minister to him as well.

I am weary emotionally tonight and glad to be back in the hotel. Honestly I'm ready for this all to be **over**! But it's in God's timing. Please pray against frustration and discouragement... that Brian as well as the rest of us will continue to rejoice step by step as we see God's hand of mercy and healing. Thank you!

*** *Looking back: At this point I was still staying in a hotel room that had been provided for us by a loving family member. It was designed for a long-term stay, had a little kitchenette, comfortable bed— was a nice* *room. But it just was so strange to be there! During the daytime while at the hospital with Brian, I was—as I mentioned earlier—operating in the "take care of things mode," thinking, "OK, what needs to be done?" However, at night when I would go back to the hotel room, it was such a surreal, unusual, "not normal" experience. I just wanted to have my husband and my children, myself and my dog back at our beautiful little home! I struggled emotionally wondering how long this would go on.*

July 17, 2014 PRIVATE JOURNAL

Hebrews 4:12 (AMP)

12 For the Word that God speaks is alive and full of power [making it active, operative, energizing, and effective]; it is sharper than any two-edged sword, penetrating to the dividing line of the breath of life (soul) and [the immortal] spirit, and of joints and marrow [of the deepest parts of our nature], exposing and sifting and analyzing and judging the very thoughts and purposes of the heart.

Early this morning I got the sense to pray "living water flowing over Brian," and I think William was included in that too. Also, I was pleading the blood of Jesus and asking the Holy Spirit to take from what Jesus accomplished on the cross and apply it to them. "By His stripes we are healed." (Isaiah 53:6b NKJV) I read aloud 1Peter. Our friend Michael Link was there, and of course, Brian and William. Brian had a prophetic word for William about singing at the top of his lungs praising God, which was a huge blessing to William. We all were singing, praying, worshipping—having church right in the hospital room. So cool!

Before bed, Michael read Romans 5–6. Then Brian asked for Psalm 38 and then Job chapters 38–42 where the Lord answers Job. We also read 1 Peter 1:23–25 and then 1 Peter 2:1. We were saved for such a higher way than this corrupt world!

Brian turned to me yesterday and said, "We have no idea how much God cares for us. And we put everything on the throne except him."

July 17, 2014 PUBLIC JOURNAL

Another very full day today with hand of God and praises all around.

Stress test this am was normal. There is no damage showing on the heart, despite the bleed/stroke and mild heart attack. (Later we learned that he did **not** have a heart attack at all! It was simply elevated enzyme levels from the stress of a stroke which can mimic heart attack indicators.)

His BP is being maintained by oral meds...sooooo he is cleared to be transferred tomorrow to Winchester Rehab center on Cork Street. That is an acute rehab center where they will apparently work him 3 hours/day with speech, physical, and occupational therapy. They needed to make sure his blood pressure was stable and his heart strong enough to be able to handle the intense rehab.

I mentioned about God's setup with Brian's roommate, William. The Holy Spirit laid on my heart early this morning to sing "Amazing Grace" for him. When I got to the room, Brian was down at the stress test (and didn't come back up for a long time). William and I sat and talked about the Lord and our testimonies of how He healed us from the musician complex of performance...that music is **not** our identity! What an incredible blessing.

A little later, I was reading 1 Peter out loud. Michael Link, William, Brian, and I were in the room. Brian often commented on the scripture, and we all were crying. Lol. Bri had a prophetic word for William too at one point, and then we all were singing, praying, worshipping. So cool!

God knew exactly what my spirit needed today...to have extensive and in-depth conversations about Jesus, worship, and music.

Thank you all for the prayers and keep it up! God is at work!

*** *Looking back, it seemed perfectly natural and seamless to be ministering to Brian's roommate, reading scripture out loud in our little room and having Bible studies together. I'm sure it did not seem normal to*

many of the staff! I can see now how it was just one more way the Lord
kept our focus on Him during this difficult time—which, of course, made
all the difference in the world!

July 18, 2014

Brian's BP spiked this morning right as the transport team was ready to
take him to Winchester. It lowered immediately but the rehab center had
freaked out by then and are postponing the transfer. Please pray against
any work of the enemy that is preventing this next step. We stand on the
power and perfect timing of Jesus Christ! Head doctor here is communicating with head doctor there to assure Brian is stable and medically safe
for transport. Thanks!

July 18, 2014 later

There are several aspects of this experience which remind me of March
28, 1997 when Garrett was born...his diagnosis of Down's syndrome
totally rocked my world. However, Jesus was so evident and reminded
me that nothing happens to us surprises God. Nothing moves Him from
the throne. After 24 hours of my soul doing free-falling somersaults back
then, it came to rest on Isaiah 42:16 (NIV) *"I will lead the blind by ways*
they have not known. Along unknown paths I will guide them. I will turn
the darkness into light before them and make the rough places smooth.
These are the things I will do. I will not forsake them."

Something else we learned on Garrett's journey is that we now walk
a path which many others walk on as well. We have entrance into a world
of experiences and a slice of life which we otherwise would not have
known. There are beautiful people here, fragrant life, vibrant joy to the
glory of God. You can google "Welcome to Holland" essay. It expresses
it beautifully. (See Appendix.)

It is the same with this. Before seven days ago, I really had never
thought about strokes or the effect they have on families. Now we have
access into a whole new community of people. Interesting journey. And

although it is certainly not one we would have chosen, it is one the Lord has seen fit to allow. We trust Him, and we are seeing Him work.

Unlike with Garrett, this is something from which we fully expect Brian to recover. But it will still allow us to relate and to minister to a whole different group of people.

July 18, 2014 again

Funds have already come in and I just want to say how much we appreciate it! I cannot imagine the tab that we are racking up... ambulance, helicopter, all kinds of tests, five days in ICU at $637/day, now rehab at about the same out of pocket cost... oh, well. It doesn't matter. I got Brian's last paycheck from work yesterday, but we know God will provide. We are incredibly blessed. Thank you!

And I came home exhausted last night to a beautifully clean house and a new toilet installed thanks to friends from our church. Thanks so much!

Brian turned to me at one point yesterday afternoon after we had been listening to some worship on Pandora. He said, " We have no idea how much God cares for us. And yet, we place everything on the throne above him."

Yep. True words. But we can choose to make Him first.

July 19, 2014

Thank you for praying about the perfect timing for Brian's transfer to Winchester Rehab yesterday. It was a long, interesting day. After the BP spike and the transport hold at 11:30 AM, the head doctors chatted and transport came back at 5:00 PM. In the meantime, we had some more great fellowship with his roommate, William. God also had someone else for me to encourage....

I felt led to walk down to the chaplain's office. I really didn't want to because I didn't feel like talking to anyone, plus I knew I would just sit there and cry. But I thought if I could find a piano, it would be wonderful to sit, play, and worship for a while. No piano, but had a nice cry/chat with the chaplain. The Lord had me share testimony of the praises. Then she shared a personal request, so we prayed together. If Brian had left before noon, that wouldn't have happened. Basically, God rocks!

I am home today and Brian is getting evaluated to begin the intense therapy up in Winchester. Please be praying that his BP would lower and stabilize, and that his heart would be strong for the workout he is embarking on. Thank you!

*** *Looking back, although it was encouraging that he was ready to be transferred to rehab, it was also an odd realization—life is not going to just go back to "normal." This journey is far from over. Now he won't be in the hospital, but actually a rehab center...for how long? What does this mean for our lives? My schedule? My work? Our children? Despite standing on my faith in the promises of God for full recovery, it felt very strange to now have to navigate this new step. Again God's strength is made perfect in weakness, and I needed to trust Him and take one day at a time, sometimes one hour at a time.*

RESIDENTIAL REHAB

July 21, 2014

Chuck and Wanda are up with Brian today. Family is allowed to participate in his rehab. On my heart this morning has been to pray for the Lord's strength to be given to Brian's left side especially. Also, pray for us as we watch—it is **not** easy to see him like this. **But** we must fix our eyes on Jesus **and** recount the miracles that have **already** been accomplished this last ten days! And there are more to come, we know!

My prayer for several days has been, "Lord, I ask that in your mercy this trial would be as short as possible while still accomplishing everything you desire."

Complete and total healing and restoration in the name and power of Jesus Christ we know are coming!

Thanks for your prayers on the journey.

July 20, 2015

Brian: Being still…

This was one thing God showed me as I started to go through this process, especially when I got to rehab. Things were a little calmer because I was out of the woods health wise—now we just had to deal with this. God showed me just to be still, showed me how to focus on the quietness and just listen. When you're in that situation, especially when something traumatic has happened in your life, people want to throw stuff at you—information, give you activities, everybody wants to keep you up to date on what is going on etc. So there are many of things coming at you at once. Even so, you're still left with hours of nothing to do.

I really didn't have the desire to watch TV for hours, or even turn it on. Consequently, what do you do? You lie there in bed. You spend hours just thinking. That could drive a person nuts, but God really showed me how to just be still in Him. Even though this was a trauma in my life, the blessing was that I was just abiding in Him right now. Nothing else. I couldn't do anything else—couldn't get up and go visit with anybody or even hang out at the cafeteria. (Not only was I extremely limited in movement, but mentally I couldn't handle a lot of noise and stimulation either.) So God was teaching me how to be able to rest in Him even when people would start bombarding me with activities and information. I was present and paying attention, but I was able to disconnect and just abide in Him. I realized this: "All this stuff really isn't what matters. What matters is my relationship with God. Am I listening?"

I don't think I ever really had that before. The World was always pushing me—"You need to take care of this...you need to work on this project, do this or do that, go here or there, make this happen" —things were constantly pulling me or pushing me. That's not God. He doesn't force. He doesn't push. He quietly moves you along; He makes you want to be with Him. Not out of some obligation. In the rehab center I learned how to *not* be led by the world! It's a weird feeling!

Now two years after I'm out of rehab, and I'm living in Texas...but I don't feel like I'm being pulled in any direction. Yes there are moments that I think, "Well I'd like to be able to do such and such again." But then I think, "No, I'm just going to wait until God lets me know. I realize my flesh wants to do _____, but what does God want me to do?" I'll wait until He lets me know. Like working at The Drugstore (our friends' restaurant here which is one of the main attractions in town)—working there is not anything my flesh would ever want to do. I never knew anything about working at a restaurant, and that was never anything which appealed to me. But our friends wanted me there, largely because they wanted me to pray and be a representation of Christ there. And I felt the Lord was nudging me to do it. So I go in a couple days/week. It gets me out of the house, gives me something to do.

But really, it's ministering to people. How do I take that peace that I've found and share it with people? My message right now is this: Don't react to the world. Interact with God and He will show you how to respond. Don't respond out of the flesh. You will find the "peace that passes all understanding" when you rest in Christ. (Philippians 4:6) You don't have to partake in the drama of everyday life. I'm starting to understand what it means to be "in the world but not of it."

July 22, 2014

Just some info about visiting because I know there are so many people who want to see him … Winchester Rehab has visiting hours Mon–Fri 4:00–9:00 PM, Sat noon—9:00 PM and Sunday 10:00 AM–9:00 PM. No kids under twelve are allowed; they would need to wait downstairs because as soon as you get off the elevator on the third floor, you are in the unit with patient rooms.

He is in an intense rehab program, doing therapy about 3 hours/day. As you can imagine with any brain injury, he gets really tired! So at this time it's probably best to limit visits to about 15 minutes in his room. If I am there or his parents are, we can go downstairs or take a walk and visit longer. But at this point, sleep is very restorative and we want Brian to be able to rest when he needs to. Thank you for understanding! We truly appreciate the love and support!

I am heading up this afternoon to participate in his therapy. They welcome family members to come and be involved since we will be helping him once he gets home as well.

Brian:

In residential rehab, someone would come into my room to help me get to the restroom, get dressed, brush my teeth, learn how to shave again, and take me down to breakfast in the wheelchair. Then I would go down to the big physical therapy area for 2 hours. Afterwards, I'd come back to my bed and sleep for 3–4 hours because it would totally wipe me out physically and mentally. (The brain is the main thing affected by a stroke, so any stimulation is heightened. Even little things that we would not even think about can be overwhelming for someone with a brain injury—visual as well as audio stimulation, TV, lots of people around, movement— all these things your brain has to process. Easy for the normal brain, totally exhausting for an injured brain.) As I grew stronger, I'd have a couple more hours of therapy in the afternoon as well.

Now looking back on this I see...moment of the stroke was like salvation. I didn't die; it was like I was reborn. This was a physical parallel to our spiritual existence. God was showing me how we're like that. We're born into Christ, but we don't know how to do anything because we've never been there before. God said, "This journey is very much like your faith. I saved you from death, and you're forever saved. But now how much you get back has to do with how much you want to put into it. I'm not talking about faith by works—the stroke happened and it stopped. So it was over. But now how much I grew in usefulness was up to me. Was I going to be content to say, "I had a stroke and I'm on disability now... I can sit on the couch and watch TV all day? Or do I want to grow in Christ, so can be spiritually used by Him?" He lets us decide that!

July 20, 2014

We continue to be blessed by all the love and support of family and friends far and near through messages, prayers, cards, money, food, and offers of any help we need. Thank you so much!

I am sitting here while Brian snores in his room at rehab. The boys were here with me for a few minutes and now are headed out. His roommate is an older man who has a loud TV as his constant companion. Pray for me because I don't like TV, especially when it is blaring nonsense not of my choosing. I think the nurse just turned it down, praise the Lord!

Brian has had several visitors just today already, so he is pretty tired. I'm going to read him some scripture…he wants to hear the writings of Paul. Miss you, William. Wish you were here listening.

Report yesterday was that he took a couple steps while holding onto a railing in the hallway! Yeah! Got the glasses back on because he is struggling a bit with double vision.

Our church had service in the park this morning. It was a blessing to lead worship with our dear friends! God is good and He is worthy of praise! That is because of Who He is, not determined by circumstances. Bryan Patrick offered a strong message of encouragement that "love believes the best!" Amen!

Lord, continue to do your best in and through Brian because You are Love.

*** *Looking back, I remember going to church that morning. I thought I was doing pretty well. However, when I stepped into a "normal life" experience and saw people, heard conversations about everyday things, it brought quickly into focus that we were not at all in a normal life experience at that point. This was a very difficult reality check—felt rather like a slap in the face or a sudden jolt from a sound sleep. I wanted to just reenter that normal world—that we had been ingrained and functioning in until just days before. Couldn't I just wake up from this traumatizing dream and get back to normal life with my husband healthy and standing by my side? Let's just think about grocery shopping or the schedule for the week instead of how many steps he was able to walk without the wheelchair! Of course that is not possible, so you just keep putting one foot in front of the other, leaning on God's strength (because you certainly have none of your own left) and move forward.*

July 22, 2014

The reality is hitting me that this is potentially a long process, although I also believe that God **is** doing a quick work and can instantly heal him!

I was here for his physical, occupational, and speech therapy, and they were noticing more strength and muscle reaction than even yesterday. Praise God! I keep reminding myself where we were a week ago—in ICU hooked to IV BP drip. So we have lots to be thankful for!

The speech therapist said since his stroke was on the right side (which controls the left side), she needs to check cognitive skills, abstract reasoning, memory. He breezed right through all of that, teasing her and cracking jokes throughout. It was so good to hear him laugh!

July 23, 2014

For anyone else like me who really does not like to exercise all that much—it is a necessary thing but not really what I would call "fun"—I will pass along a challenge I received this morning from the Holy Spirit, Who is good at giving those if we choose to listen.

My husband will work for hours today just to regain muscle strength to move the left side of his body. There is nothing wrong with my whole body—except laziness—therefore I really have no excuse to not exercise!

So I did.

Word from his parents, who were with him today, is that he had another good day. He slept right through lunch being tired from the morning therapy, but his speech therapist was bringing him some orange sherbet at 3:00 PM when I called. He's good. lol

July 24, 2014 Morning

We have been Discover Card holders and customers in good standing for over twenty-five years, and yet there is no program by which they can defer payment in this kind of situation. **But** the manager I was speaking with in Ohio quoted scripture to me and said she stands with me in full faith that Brian will be completely healed and restored in the name of Jesus Christ. "By his stripes we are healed." She said he is already healed in the spiritual realm; we just haven't seen it in the natural realm yet. I have been saying that very thing today more than once. God just makes me laugh sometimes. Thank you, Father.

Working through paperwork of financial aid applications for the hospitals as well as temporary disability and Medicaid for Brian. Appreciate prayers for favor and quick processing. We continue to see how the Lord is our Provider, and we are so blessed and humbled at the gifts we have received.

I will be heading up to participate in Brian's therapy again today; looking forward to more encouraging reports! Colton is at work, and Garrett is going to the new *Planes* movie with Nana and Pop.

July 24, 2014 Evening

I spent the afternoon with Brian again today.

He was able to take several steps today using a claw-type cane and support from the therapists. He's able to kind of swing his left leg to take steps. He said it feels weird, kind of like when your leg has fallen asleep. He also has a little bit of numbness on his left side of his mouth, lips…you can pray about that. The therapists are very surprised that he has not lost any cognitive skills, memory, or abstract reasoning, etc. They said that is unusual, as is the fact that he never lost consciousness throughout this whole ordeal. Praise God!

Brian told the speech therapist that he feels like he has a hat on his head, and he keeps reaching to take it off. Later, on speaker phone with a friend, we shared this with her. I was reminded how I prayed for him Tuesday, "In the name of Jesus Christ of Nazareth, rise up and walk!" She said when she had heard that, she thought of "Lazarus, come forth!" And what happened when he came forth? They had to unwrap the grave clothes. So we prayed to that affect, while I mimed the "unwrapping" motion around his head. I will be very fascinated to see what the Lord does from this.

Aimee Patrick has been such a blessing helping me wade through paperwork and applications. She was checking online with Anthem. For the helicopter ride she saw figures of $16,000 and one that said $41,000. And she saw one bill for INOVA that said $87,000! I just laughed! I can't wait to see how the Lord is going to provide with all of this. Aimee is helping me fill out paperwork for Medicaid for Brian, SSI and SSDI for Garrett and Brian, and financial aid for the two hospitals. Please keep those matters in prayer. We know that the Lord is our Provider, and we know He has a special plan in this matter!

July 24, 2014
Brian had a surprise visit from a couple therapy dogs, two beagles, Baxter and Buster. Not as great as Zeppelin, but still sweet.

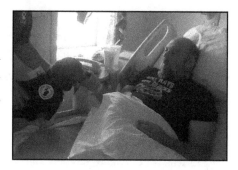

July 25, 2014
I just want to say **thank you** again to all of you who have made financial donations to us during this time. Some of them I know; many are anonymous. We have received cards with checks in them, cash pressed into a hand meant for us, and contributions on the caring website. Please know that we are so humbled and grateful! The Lord is our Provider, and He is showing us how He provides through the Body of Christ. After all, it's all His $$ anyway. He owns the cattle on a thousand hills. He's my heavenly Father, and He ain't broke. Thank you again.

From an article my cousin shared on Facebook—

Great quote from Kara Tippetts' blog called Mundane Faithfulness:

"My life may not be written as I had dreamed, but that does not mean that it is not good. Hard is not the absence of God's goodness. And those that would tell you it is haven't looked deeply upon Jesus. They know little of his abiding grace, and simply think health and wealth are the only signs of the faithfulness of Jesus. That is a weak God, and simply not the truth of the gospel. Look closely how Jesus redeemed you. It isn't pretty, but it is

good. So good. Then why oh why do we grieve so deeply when our story is written in hard? Simply, we are weak. We long for comfort and easy. I'm the first one in that line. But cancer and walking this 'hard' has taught me something better."

Yep. Once again, reminded me of the "Welcome to Holland" essay in relation to life with a special needs child. (See Appendix)

July 26, 2014

I'm looking forward to seeing my hubby today! I so miss him!

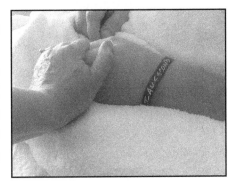

I passed the baton back to Brian today…told him I sensed this morning that it was time he wear the bracelet and use it as a conversation tool with his therapists.

Bryan Patrick posted this on July 26, 2014:

Aim and I visited Brian today and while we were talking the nurse suggested we might like to take him outside on the big patio, but we would have to sign him out before we went. Brian then turns to me with a laugh, saying, "I'm like a puppy at the pet store. You have to sign me out. I'm a big ferocious puppy." Yeah, I'd say our brother is definitely on the mend.

July 26, 2014

Bri is doing well today. I was surprised to see how much he could move his left arm and leg compared to just the other day. He says he feels strength returning, just doesn't feel he has control of his limbs yet. The double vision is almost gone! Praise God! We are so grateful and encouraged! Enjoyed a visit in the patio today with precious longtime friends whom we met our first month in Virginia in our little tiny house on the mountain with the cistern. Great memories and an encouragement to see them.

July 27, 2014

It was tough going to church today without Brian ... knowing he wouldn't be with me and wouldn't be playing guitar. I felt teary all morning so I collapsed into a friend's arms when I walked in the door. I went back to pray with the guest worship team and had another emotional breakdown. I said to another friend, "I don't know why I can't have an emotional breakdown in the privacy of my own home." She said, "Then we wouldn't get to love on you." Yes ... true. Had lots of love and prayers, as well as Spirit-filled worship and Word, and I felt **much** encouraged a couple hours later.

Enjoyed some quiet time with Brian this afternoon/evening. The boys and I wheeled him out to the patio for an hour. After the boys left, we came inside. Then the tech turned off the bed alarm (it's very sensitive to alert them if he tries to get out of bed on his own)—but he turned it off so I was able to curl up in bed with him! We took a nap cuddled together which was wonderful ... until his roommate's alarm of some sort started blaring. But it was good.

July 28, 2014 posted by Bryan Patrick:

Just now leaving from visiting Brian. I came to encourage but leave encouraged. I'm not surprised. God is ministering to, and through, my brother.

July 28, 2014

Colton has been such a great helper and support during these last couple weeks! Tonight I got Garrett his favorite chicken (from Walmart) and for Colton and me ... marinated steak and fresh veggies cooked on the grill! Yummmm. Hurry home, Colt, it smells good!

I received encouragement from John, one of Brian's closest friends, today. He has been brainstorming things to keep Brian's mind engaged and to keep him from being bored when he is not doing therapy—a large print Bible, or Bible on CD, portable DVD player, a notebook to record some thoughts, prayers, or goals, or to make notes on what the Lord is saying to him during this time. All great ideas, and I will discuss them with Bri tomorrow!

He also encouraged me that there are many creative ways to adjust our home for a temporary time while Brian recuperates. Also very true, and I know I have people standing in line waiting to be told what we need. Thank you! I want to talk to the therapists this week to see what skills they look for him to have before he can come home.

I was honest with John that I was having a hard time. I'm ready for this all to be over. But he reminded me to take one day at a time, said he and Brian had specifically prayed about that yesterday. He said, "Sheila, many women lose their precious husbands from a stroke. At least you have him; and his personality, sense of humor, cognitive skills are all very much intact. That is something to be truly thankful for! Oftentimes with a stroke that is not the case. You have your sweet husband, your best friend, and you know that God doesn't waste anything. God is working many wonderful things during this time." **So true**! I thanked him for the words of encouragement. I needed that renewed perspective today.

God is so faithful! He hears our heart cries and answers.

July 31, 2014

We are ready to start afternoon therapy. Brian just told me that when he woke up this morning, he could wiggle his fingers and toes a little bit on the left side! Yeah! Today is the third week mark.

*** *Boy! Looking back I think, "The three week mark." We have now passed the three-year mark! I'll admit that at times I still struggle, wanting all of this to be over! And yet along the way in the process you discover a "new normal." The process in and of itself is the journey. The goal of life is not just arriving at a destination, but is learning "joy on the journey" to quote a phrase I remember hearing as a kid in the 70s.*

Later on July 31, 2014

Here's a big surprise...Italian food is my comfort food. So tonight I decided to treat myself to Olive Garden and then come back to spend a couple more hours with Brian. I was feeling kind of lonely, but figured it'd be "me and God" for dinner.

When I sat down I looked to my right—and I knew the lady at the next table. She gave me a hug and said she was praying for Brian. The waiter was very kind and I shared why I was there alone. He said he would say a prayer for me...also that he lost his spouse two years ago. I ordered my favorite—the "Tour of Italy"—and told him I would take Brian the leftovers.

He packed up my leftovers for me and gave me a free dessert. Then he said, "There is no bill. I told the managers what was going on, and we wanted your dinner to be on us. We know everything will continue to go well with your husband." I was so touched and of course instantly burst into tears (which sort of freaked my sweet waiter man out). The manager then came and sat down and chatted with me, again expressing compassion and their good wishes and prayers. I have always highly recommended Olive Garden, but will even more so now.

Truly I was overwhelmed by such kindness from total strangers. But I also know it was the Lord just showing me that He was watching over me...and blessing me (us)! Thank you, Father!

Leaving Olive Garden I saw a young couple on the side of the room apparently arguing. I wanted to go over and tell them to appreciate each other, work it out and be thankful!

When I got home tonight from being with Brian most of the day, I realized that I hadn't paid for anything all day! For lunch, I used a Subway gift card we received this week. (There's a Subway one block from the rehab center). Dinner was the beautiful Olive Garden story. Filled up with gas at Sheetz with a gift card from another friend today, and got a few groceries with food stamps we qualified for due to the situation. God provides!

August 1, 2014

The following is a text I received from one of our prayers warriors:

Up early this morning and instructed to pray for the miraculous for Brian. So I asked the Lord, "How do I do that?" He had me look up the word "miraculous." It means, "The nature of a miracle performed by a supernatural power." Well, we know that that is Him! A miracle is to affect the physical world, which surpasses all known or natural powers, with the supernatural.

*So I asked God to affect Bri's physical world with His supernatural power. To bring about a sign and wonder for His glory. I'm not sure what this is all about yet, but God is up to **something** more than our understanding knows or what we can see.*

Isaiah 35:6 (NLT) says "The lame will leap like a deer, and those who cannot speak will sing for joy!"

Amen! I receive that, Lord! Have your way!!

August 1, 2014

Each morning as I am waking up, I often will ask the Lord what He wants me to pray for Brian that day. Today I got the answer: TRUTH.

The Bible study we were having moments before stroke occurred 7/10 was on the verse John 14:6 (NIV, emphasis mine) where Jesus is saying, *"I AM the Way, the Truth and the Life. No man comes to the Father except through me."*

Lord I pray that your Truth would wash all over Brian today! The Truth of Who you are. The True perspective of this situation—that this is only a test. God is in control, on the throne and glorified. Our job is to surrender. Let the Truth of your healing power, Jesus, completely consume Brian from the top of his head to the tips of his toes. And I do pray that full motion, movement, and control would return soon. Any fear is a **lie** from the enemy and I bind that in the name of Jesus. (Anyone who has been around Brian in Bible study the last year or so has heard him talk about the "lie" ... if you haven't, ask him about it!)

We welcome and seek after and only desire Your Truth, Lord God! And thank you, Jesus, that You ARE Truth.

A comment from a friend: John 8:31–32 (NKJV), *"If you abide in My word, you are My disciple indeed. And you shall know the the truth, and the truth shall make you free!!"* Father, we pray that Your Truth will set Brian free—from every chain, from every infirmity, from all that seeks to kill, steal, and destroy, and that every and any stronghold be broken in the Name of Jesus! Let this resting time be a time of strengthening and abiding in You as never before! And may it make him abide in the Truth that sets Brian free in his heart, body, and mind fully healed, fully restored, and glorified for Your glory!!

*** Looking back as I write this, now three-plus years after the stroke, the promise of this previous paragraph has been realized in our lives! Even though he still has some physical deficits he has been amazingly restored, and time of rest has indeed been a time of strengthening and abiding in the Lord as never before. And in fact, now (January 2018 at this writing) we see how the Lord has and is using it as preparation for the next adventure He has for us!

August 1, 2014

Brian said to me yesterday, "When people are going through hard times, they often think, 'Well, I am going to praise the Lord because then He will bless me and I will be healed.' What I am realizing is that we just need to praise the Lord. Period. Not because we are hoping to get something, but because He is worthy. That's not easy to do. But that is what I am trying to do and what we need to do in this time."

He continued, "Yes, I do believe that I will be healed. The Lord has told me that this is a season. However, I do not know the duration or the details of that season. But really it doesn't matter because it's all about God. He is God. I am not. He has told me He has purpose in this. I am praising Him. Period."

I told him at some point I would like to video him saying this and share it with you. It is even more powerful hearing it from his slurred speech and from his wheelchair. Have I mentioned how much I love this man? Or how much I love what God is doing in and through Him?

BRIAN: reflecting about friends...
In a time like this, you learn who your friends are, the people who really are close to you. For example, my dear friend John...I'd been beside him when he was having a rough time emotionally. We played music together on worship team at church, but he didn't go to church the whole time I was in rehab. He would come up there and we would study together. He said he didn't want to play without me. That touched me. I realized what a close friend he was. I was always the person who tried to be there for others. I was always the strong one. I hadn't needed to call people. Now I was stuck in a bed, pushed around in a wheelchair. My friend John showed me he was there for me.

Another friend, Michael Link, came to see me too...made me laugh, encouraged me. He said he kept waiting to hear from God to punch me in the stomach and "Bang!" I'd be healed. But I told him I didn't think I was supposed to be healed instantly. It's in this process I have learned so much about myself and God—how I see God.

There were some concepts spiritually that I had wrong—we all have. We try to make it too complicated. It's a simple faith, a simple fact that God loves us. He loves us so much he couldn't leave us in the state we're in. He left heaven and came. We just have to believe in that and enter into a relationship. Jesus Christ accomplished everything on the cross. We try to take something back and think we have to accomplish it. When you're lying on a bed and realize you can't accomplish anything right now, then you realize you really never could!

August 2, 2014

Last night was "date night." Aimee and I cooked dinner, met Bryan Patrick, and ate out in the patio with Brian. I meant to take a picture as we had a tablecloth, candles, and everything! He hadn't shaved, though! He said they worked him hard at Occupational Therapy , but they didn't do the shaving. Oh, well. It was a very nice evening eating good food, talking, laughing, praying, and getting into some deep discussions about the Word and the Lord.

When I got home I learned that my sweet daddy is probably going to see Jesus very soon. Please pray for God's perfect timing in light of Brian's potential release date, etc.

And thank you again to those who have made financial donations on the WeCare website or personally or through the mail. We are humbled and amazed to see how the Lord provides for us through the Body of Christ!

I'm up early this morning, so heading out to the studio for some worship time. Interesting that Colton fell asleep on the couch in here last night instead of in his bed in the studio. Gives me some privacy.

August 2, 2014

Thank you all for your love and support during this time! I know many of you are itching to cook us meals, etc. Believe me I will take you up on that when Brian gets home! But for now we are running different directions and eating out one to two meals a day most days.

Something else we will likely need when he gets home, as I will be resuming a fairly full teaching schedule, is someone to be with him sometimes in the house while I am in the studio. Brian-sitting! Lol. However, we do anticipate that he will really be fairly self-sufficient in pretty short order. He can already do many transfers with wheelchair almost unassisted.

*** *In the process of going back over these journals to write the book, I commented that he always was so kind, so pleasant through the therapies.*

48

He never seemed to get angry or frustrated, which was and is amazing to me.

BRIAN said,
I feel like I had made my peace with the situation. I had peace with God in the ambulance that night. I died to self that night. Yes, you do that when you get saved, but we really don't do it. We keep trying to keep some of ourselves. But that night I died. I figured, "Anything after this is gravy. There's nothing I can do. I can't make myself get up." It's not like I could just work hard to recover from a broken ankle.

So in my mind I figured I need to take each day as it came, and it's all just about what God gives me back. It's whatever he wants me to have the ability to do. Sure, I want to be totally back, or to never have had this happen in the first place! I had hours to myself— yes, I would pray and plead asking the Lord to have my hand back, let me be able to walk, all these things one naturally wants back. People would say, "You need to claim that in the name of the Lord, take that healing, pray without ceasing!" I would think, what else is there to say than what I have already said?

I'm alone with my God in a hospital bed. I think, "God, You know. I can't presume to tell You anything. You hold all creation in the palm of Your hand. You know my heart and I want to be healed. But I also know what You've shown me through the Word and spiritually that we need to be obedient to Your will. When and if it's Your will that I be healed, I will be healed. I can't get You to change your mind, and if You have purpose, then I wouldn't want you to change Your mind."

I am a child of God. I am His instrument on this earth. He saved me from death in that ambulance. I don't know why. He has a reason, and He'll let me know. Surrendering...means also surrendering my claim to being healed, surrendering my claim to anything. Why do we assume hearing that "in Christ you're healed" means physically? Yes, I am healed— spiritually and eternally! And certainly God can and often does heal physically as well. But I believe that is not the most important type of healing.

Looking back *now after two years, I realize I've been able to talk to so many people that I would have never had anything in common with before. How many people through various therapy sessions got to hear about God? We always proclaimed God, kept good attitudes; that was unique because so many people get frustrated, get mean because they have no hope.*

Someone at work said to me the other day, "Oh, I could just kill you!" I said, "I've tried that ... it doesn't scare me anymore." God let me go right to the edge and look over the edge of death, but it has no teeth because of Jesus. I have to believe in the promises—I have no fear of death. There are things I like, things I want to do, but that's all flesh. As Paul says it's all dung compared to Christ! So why do we wish for dung? (See Philippians 3:8 KJV)

August 3, 2014

On the way to therapy yesterday afternoon with Brian, he was anxious to show his occupational therapist the "new gift" he had received that morning—more extension in his fingers and the ability to squeeze a little tighter with his hand. She was delighted and kept remarking how amazed at how quickly he has been regaining strength! I said, "Lots of people are praying!"

Brian says every morning he wakes up and finds a "new gift"— something he is able to do that he wasn't the day before. Praise God! It is incredible to watch how God is working.

Even in the times (like last evening) when I am just bone tired, I stand in wonder at the awesomeness of the Jesus we serve. Please keep praying!

*** *Looking back, yes I remember those times that I was just incredibly tired. Exhausted to the point of desperation and not knowing how I would take another step. It was in those moments I was acutely aware of Jesus literally holding me, sustaining me. The Bible says the Word is our life, our very breath. We can realize in times of difficulty that those phrases are not hyperbole or metaphor. They are truth!*

August 3, 2014

My sweet daddy stepped into eternity Saturday around 3:00 PM at age 98 ½ very peacefully and with my mother at his side. Thank you for the prayers. Services will be next weekend in New Castle, Pennsylvania, so I will leave Virginia Friday. My father was a kind, loving man of faith and integrity. Among his many gifts were laughter and making people feel welcome. I will miss him but am so grateful he is now completely at peace. And what amazing things must he be seeing and experiencing now!

Dad at twenty-one years of age (1937) and also in New Guinea during WWII

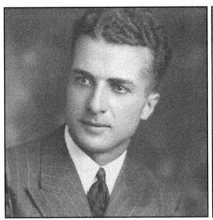 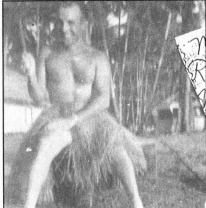

August 4, 2014

Brian continues to make improvements every day! His spirits and sense of humor are great. Praise the Lord.

Prayer points: his BP is good but he is on a lion's load of meds. He still has some numbness in his lips. And he still kind of feels like there is a warm towel around his neck/head. (I imagine this is the blood and swelling still on his brain.)

He is very anxious to come home! And although we miss him terribly and are weary with the routine, I also want him to get as much benefit as possible from the 4 hours of personal attention with therapists each day. He has good stamina and a great work ethic; therefore they are pouring effort and time into him—as much as he can tolerate! Just pray for the Lord's perfect timing in all that.

I won't be able to go see him as much this week. I appreciate your prayers for me as well…as I resume music camp and piano lessons and then head to Pennsylvania Friday afternoon for my dad's funeral.

Thank you!

August 6, 2014

Sitting here with a mug of hot cocoa—I guess I'm carrying on my dad's addiction. Reflecting on a long day. Sorting out screwups with Social Security in the midst of music camp. (Yes, I did the alliteration purposely.) Laid down for a brief window in the afternoon, which was interrupted by issues with Anthem. Aimee Patrick to the rescue on that one, again! Thank you! After teaching a few lessons, I headed up to have dinner with a "soul mate" friend—thank you for the girl-time fellowship! Then finally I walked in (well, dragged in, really) to see my hubby.

His excitement to see me wiped away my weariness, and what he showed me did so even more—he is able to squeeze my hand with his left hand! He said, "I'm not going to crush anyone's hand yet, but I can do it."

During therapy today, Brian said they had him on his stomach, then propping himself up on his elbow and then on all fours (hands and knees). He was able to support himself and could even lift up his strong arm so that his left one was supporting his weight! I can't wait to take some videos in therapy tomorrow and share them.

Praise God! That was quite a gift today!

Since I hadn't seen him for a few days, I had several cards to share with him, as well as a present we received. Together we opened cards and once again were humbled to find checks and gift cards. Thank you! It is humbling to receive. We appreciate it and look forward to the day when we will be able to give back.

Brian asked for prayer that his brain would get clearer and that the swelling (and blood) would go back to normal. He said he feels like his thoughts are kind of "jumpy"—it's hard to concentrate for very long. He also wants to have more control of his right hand, so that he can write better and record his thoughts cohesively. I was somewhat surprised because he certainly seems to be thinking and processing clearly. He said the "hat" that he felt around his head feels like it is smaller. He also describes it as a "towel." To me those are descriptions of the blood and the swelling. I speak to that in the name of Jesus and say, "Shrink!"

Thank you for praying!

August 10, 2014
Facebook post from Sheila on August 10th:
My dad, Ralph Mooney, Jr., died last Saturday at 98 1/2 years of age. He had been in a nursing home for two months. Colton and I are in Pennsylvania this weekend for his memorial service. We had visitation at the funeral home yesterday from 2:00–5:00 PM and then an honor guard at 5:00 PM with full military honors as a sendoff. (He was in WWII, rose to the rank of first lieutenant, Army Corps of Engineers, in the South Pacific Theater.) Very meaningful. Today is the service at 2:30 PM. The Lord made clear to me He wanted me to sing two songs I wrote, so you can keep me in prayer. My mom is doing quite well, although of course she is tired.

Brian continues to make very good progress. It is likely he will come home next Friday. I'm going to ask Aimee Patrick to coordinate meals at that time, probably two to three nights per week. I'll see how much assistance Brian will need at that time. I will be teaching Tuesdays and

Wednesdays in August; he might need some people to keep him company and assist him during those days.

It has been difficult to have this with my dad at the same time, but really it has been a good break to be here with my family. They are wonderful, all believers in Christ, upbeat and encouraging. We laugh, cry, and catch up. I am so blessed. Dad had been really declining in the last year and it was stressful as my mother (eighty-one) was caring for him 24/7 until end of May. Now we know he is at peace, and she is adjusting as well. We'll get home tonight and then I can focus on Brian. God's timing.

August 11, 2014

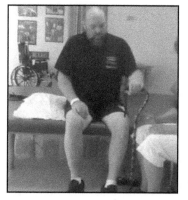

Brian jokingly asked one of his best friends and car buddies to bring him a Hurst shifter to practice with instead of this cane!

It has certainly been a rough month with Brian's stroke and my dad's failing health and ultimate home-going last weekend. I have cried more publicly than ever in my life.

Several people at the services this weekend asked me, "How are you holding up?" I answered, "The Lord." I don't mean that to sound glib or trite. We often quote scriptures about God's strength being our refuge. In fact, my dad's favorite verse was Nahum 1:7 (NIV) which says, *"The Lord is good, a refuge in times of trouble. He cares for those who trust in Him."* We don't realize how true that is until we hit times like this.

A friend/mentor said to me recently, "People look at something like what you are going through, and they expect you to fall apart like the world would fall apart. But you are not citizens of the world. You are citizens of the Kingdom!" True! And we have a King who not only loves us, paid the penalty for us, but Who also carries and sustains us.

That's the only way I am functioning right now. Jesus. And that is something that is available to every living soul on the planet!

Please do not misunderstand or think that I don't appreciate your concern and kind words! They have been part of the sustaining! But I want to be clear on the Source.

Today we had a 40-minute break in-between therapies so we went out on the patio. Then we turned to go back inside. There was a little lady sitting nearby. I had seen her a few times walking on the patio, usually with cute hats, very, very thin. Today I said hello and asked how long she has been here. She said two weeks. I asked if she knew how long she would be here ... she said, "I'm here for the duration. I won't be going home. I'm in hospice." Bri and I moved over and talked with her a few minutes. My dad's death gave me an opening to share with her. I asked her if she has peace about the next stage of the journey, and she said she does. We talked a little while and ended up praying for her. God appointments ... so neat.

Brian's testimony:
Recorded on August 11, 2014 on the patio of the rehab center. His speech was still rather slurred.

Sheila: Do you want to just say what you remember from the thing in general?

Brian: Well, I can remember that when I had the stroke we were talking in the studio about Job. We were talking about how Job had to learn that God is just God. To some He gives and to some He takes away. (Job 1:20 NIV) That does not detract from Who God is. He is still the same God, and we need to worship Him just because of that. Not because of what we have or don't have, but just because He's God. He made everything we see or He gave us the ability to make it. He gives to some and to others He doesn't give. But He's God, so whatever He does is right.

I can remember when I got in the ambulance, in the ER, or even the helicopter ride. I was never afraid because I knew God was in control. He was either going to take me and I would slip away, or He was going to save me and restore me. If He did save me, it would be because He had a darn good reason. Because He's God. He doesn't do things without a reason.

He is restoring me. I feel I am getting better. My speech, my legs, my arm, my left side is getting stronger. He's restoring me. I'm reminded of King Nebuchadnezzar—he ate grass like a wild animal for seven years. Seven years! If we go seven days without something we feel like we're suffering. He went seven years. God restored him, but first he had to admit Who God was. He had to admit that. If you read some of those passages, notice what Nebuchadnezzar said about God when he admitted Who God was. So how could we not worship Him? How could we not be on our knees before Him? He is God. He is the Almighty Creator.

Recorded April 2017:
Brian: Reflecting on wanting to go home:
I wanted so badly to get home at that point. In my mind I think I reasoned, "If I can just get home, I will feel more normal, I can get over this." Because physically that's what I'd always done—I could get through this, get some sleep, and be better. I don't think I fully recognized that I was going home but wouldn't be able to get back to who I was right away.

NOW LOOKING BACK…two-and-a-half years out, I can see that. I didn't know it at the time. What God showed me in that time was yes, I wanted it very badly. Friends were encouraging me come back to work, trying to be nice; they had the best intentions. Now that I'm in Texas and looking back, I see more clearly. That time was when I started to realize, "I can't try to jump back in to where I was." I had to have time for God to show me how to be me again.

I need this time away to sort out who I am in Jesus. Sort out my identity from the world I had created...time alone, and just the two of us together...not my whole world of cars and music. Cars and music were what my life revolved around, and that was taken away. The harder I tried to reenter that world, the harder and more frustrating it became. So I started to realize that I needed to get away. This was a huge reason behind our move across country— besides just sensing God's call. But when it was all said and done, this reshaping of my identity was probably the biggest reason, or one of them, for sure.

While I was still in rehab, I began to think, "What am I going to DO when I get home?" In my mind I thought we'd just ease into it; I knew that's what my friends were hoping for—"It's Brian; he'll get back into it. Pretty soon he'll be back to his old self." I thought that too. That was the flesh. The spiritual side was staring to think, "Wait a minute. What's God doing? I don't want to go back to the person I was!"

*I had created a world that had revolved around **me**. God was giving me a chance in this stroke and recovery time to make my life revolve around **Him**, to reeducate myself on what is really important. He's showing us, as we truly surrender areas of our lives to Him, that He is faithful to provide the things we needed to get through the tough times. If you want to rely on your own wisdom, strength, and perseverance, He'll let you. But it's frustrating. He lets you struggle with that self-reliance because He's hoping you'll learn the lesson.*

He is still with us. We've had plenty of tough things since the stroke! But I've learned not to panic. Just stop and wait for God. He will make it work out. The world wants you to panic, start changing things around, scramble, thinking, "I've got to deal with this," or "I'm going to die, my life will be over." No! Your life is not going to come to an end because something happened. Stop. Pray about it. Read scripture. Rest on His promises that He will never leave *or forsake you. (Hebrews 13:5 NIV) He will prove that true. Just like our blowing tires in the middle of nowhere on I-10 recently. We could have panicked, but we called a local place and they said, "No problem." Why? We didn't give in to fear. We called a friend who referred us to that business. Yes, it was expensive money--wise, but money's the easiest thing for God to deal with! He owns the castle on a thousand hills! In the grand scheme of things, if the worst challenge is a $500 bill on the side of the road, then that's a small thing.*

SOME PICTURES FROM THERAPY early August 2014:

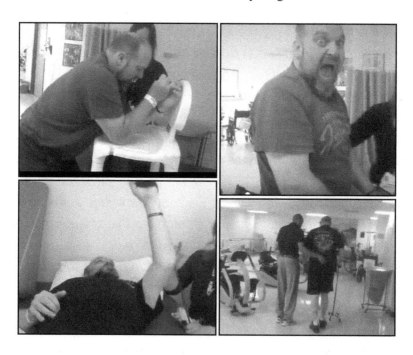

August 11, 2014

Several of you have asked me to let you know what we need. Here are some things we need in view of Brian's likely coming home date as this Friday, August 15....

1. Wheelchair with footrests (right now they are ordering one as a rental that is probably about $110/month)
2. The bars that attach to your toilet (temporarily)
3. Workout equipment so we can turn one bay of the garage into an exercise/rehab room … ex. Weight machine that is adjustable and can work both arms and legs, stationary bike, others??
4. Some 2–5 pound ankle/wrists weights

That's all I can think of for now.

Brian: Reflecting on residential therapy:
The various therapists and all the staff were terrific! The nurses who took care of me in the middle of the night were wonderful. God put people in my path. They were just caring, truly wanting to help. They were so thankful when a patient came in who really wanted to work, wanted to get better, and who wasn't angry.

I remember just watching other clients and being astounded at their rudeness to the nurses and therapists. I'd think, "These people are trying to help you and you're getting mad at them?!" I couldn't understand that. I still can't. I'm sure there's a psychological reason behind it.

Sheila: Well, they're mad at themselves, frustrated with the situation.

Brian: I just couldn't comprehend it. For me, through this whole process, sure I got frustrated. There were some anger issues at times. I'll admit I got angry with God a couple times. Then He quickly showed me, "That's not the way." But I never got angry with the people who were trying to help me … except for my wife because she lives with me and we get angry at each other sometimes. That's part of being married.

These different professionals or my friends who tried to help me, God gave me grace to see their good intentions. Also, He showed me that I was to let them help me because they needed the blessing that comes from helping others.

August 14, 2014

Leaving rehab yesterday, Brian told the staff at the front desk, "I have been here long enough to know that whatever you get paid is not enough!"

No wonder they loved him. He reminds me of my dad. One little nurse told my mom that when she went in to clean dad up, he was feeling badly that she should have to do that. He asked her name and where she lived. (Yep. That was my dad. Always asking people's names and where they were from.) Then as she was taking care of him, he just started praying out loud for her. She told mom with tears in her eyes, "I don't think anyone has ever prayed for me before." Wow.

Brian also was a great patient, showed the people respect, did what they asked him to do with 110 percent effort. He said, "I don't understand why patients complain. These folks are here to help us get better. Why would we not do what they are suggesting with a good attitude? Don't people realize that your attitude has an absolute effect on how well you recuperate?!" Nope. I guess they don't.

Brian: Then again why don't we listen to God? Christ came to heal us from the greatest problem in our lives—sin and death. He came to set us free. All He asks us to do is follow Him, lay aside our wants, admit that He's God and we're not. All we need to do is listen and obey, surrender and follow Him. We don't understand the gift of the Holy Spirit. The Spirit is here to help. Everything in us points to Jesus, or it points away from Him. Those are the only two options.

It's so much easier when we realize God wants to help us, lift us up, be with us! We try to go our own way all the time. We butt our heads up against the wall. He's God—so much bigger than a nurse or doctor! We'll listen to doctors and nurses, but we don't listen to God.

Brian's occupational therapist said he was her favorite patient ever, and she's been doing this for years. What a blessing.

A friend made homemade fudge for the therapists and the nurses, so we took that to them yesterday. Told them we'd come back to visit when Brian could play his guitar for them.

BRIAN: The night nurse and the Jesus rock story:

In Woodstock around our store-front church plant, Fresh Water Fellowship, we would often find small rocks painted gold with JESUS written on them in white. We all just came to view them as little signs of encouragement and that the Lord was with us. A friend who had a gym supported only by donations asked that a JESUS rock be given to me in rehab.

So I had this little gold rock with "JESUS" painted on it by my bed. The nurse on the night shift, around 3:00 AM, woke me to give me meds and check my blood pressure. She saw the rock and asked me about it. I said, "He is the rock on which I put my hope." She began telling me about her son who had just died in a car accident and started crying. I talked about God's sacrifice of His Son. She understood that because she would have gladly died to save her son. I said, "Yes, we all would as parents. But the difference is this: Would you have let your son die to save the world? That's what God's love represents." She couldn't comprehend it. She then told me her life story. I gave her the rock and told her to keep praying to Jesus, asking Him to reveal Himself to her…to experience a love that is big enough to sacrifice in that way.

Sure, any parent would sacrifice to save their child. God sacrificed His own Son to save the world! God's kingdom is different. Jesus knew Pilate didn't have the power. Jesus knew He had the power to raise Himself from the grave. Jesus knew death did not represent the final death! That is the illusion of this world. Our body is just a tent. Our spirit will live on forever, either with God or without God. I don't know about you, but I'd rather be with God than without God!

That was the only night I ever saw that nurse.

August 13, 2014

I woke up with the old song, "Great Is Thy Faithfulness" in my mind today. The words are so rich! My mother asked me last weekend, "Do you ever include hymns when you lead worship?" I answered, "Sometimes." A more honest answer would have been, "Rarely." She said, "You need to. They are so good." True. So get ready, worship team.

August 14, 2014 PRIVATE JOURNAL

It's been five weeks today and today Brian is coming home! I am excited and a little nervous. Things are prepared here—ramps to house and studio, twin bed in living room, equipment ready (wheelchair, four-prong cane, walker, tub/shower seat, and Aimee today is buying the rails thing that goes around the toilet.).

I'm a little concerned about handling his medications and handling him in general… **but** I must focus on Jesus and the fact that Brian is getting stronger every day. I will work myself out of a job and the equipment and ramps will eventually go away.

Lord, I am **so** very thankful that he is still here with me. And despite the difficulties, I am thankful for this season. It has been perhaps the hardest of our lives **and yet** incredibly rich in hearing Your voice and feeling. Your constant peace. What do people do who don't know You? I love You, Lord. As You have sustained us these last five weeks, so too You will sustain us now. You are the same yesterday, today, and forever.

Later that evening…

Well, it was an interesting day… a good day! The therapists gave me some last-minute instructions, Aimee got several texts asking her to grab various items from Walmart, including pizza which was Brian's request for dinner. We left rehab around 12:45 PM, drove through a Wendy's and sat in the car to eat, and then took our time driving home Route 11. It was an absolutely gorgeous day, barely 80 degrees, sunny, with a strong breeze. We talked about all kinds of things, and it was so nice to have the privacy uninterrupted. Then we waited over an hour at Walmart to fill all the meds. Friends from church were in the parking lot when we arrived, and they stood the whole time and talked with Brian while I was waiting in Walmart. That was a blessing to him and to them. They had actually been present at the Bible study in our studio when the stroke occurred, and they had been gracious, generous, and encouraging to us in many ways throughout the process.

Brian says he has prayed a lot obviously this last five weeks, and asked the Lord what he should be doing now (until he is strong enough to return to work part time). Bri said he sensed a couple ideas from the Lord but wanted to wait until God confirmed it in me. One thing was buying and reselling trucks. Doing a little bit on them before flipping them. Another was that once God gives him the ability to play guitar back, traveling around sharing testimony of what the Lord has done during this season.

We both feel strongly that we are supposed to move to Texas but have admitted to the Lord that we are a bit confused at how/when to do that in light of the recovery. We both sense that for these next couple months we need to just settle in, spend time together reading the Word, praying, being together—the Lord redeeming our time apart—and He will make clear to us the where, when, and how. We also wonder about my mother in the mix of it too, since Dad is gone now. But she also is sensing we will all receive clarity over the next couple months. I am looking forward to the time with Bri and watching to see what God will do.

Brian keeps reiterating the importance of the process. God has made that clear to him. He said while he was in ICU he couldn't really think too much, but in rehab he prayed every night and just drew close to the Lord. He was asking God if he would be totally healed, but stating that he is willing to surrender regardless. He spent much time obviously praying that through. At one point, Bri said the Lord told him, "Yes you will be completely healed. I will totally restore you. But you need to go through the process. I could instantly heal you, but then you would not have learned what I want you to learn."

*** *Looking back, I still need this reminder! The Lord is still healing Brian in many, many areas, and we continue to see benefits from "the process!" It confirms to me once again that the Lord works on multiple levels, multiple facets, not just in a one-dimensional field. As humans we tend to think more one-dimensionally with our primary goal in mind. I'm thankful that the Lord's strategies are infinitely better than mine.*

Coming Back Home

August 15, 2014

Look who's home!

After five weeks in the hospital and rehab, Brian was discharged yesterday. We are making some adjustments and getting acclimated.

We have all the equipment we need, thank the Lord, 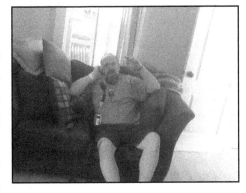 through loans and donations. He is excited to start working out, so we'll need to get moving on the work out equipment and redoing the one bay of the garage!

Thanks for your prayers! Keep them coming.

His attitude and perspective continue to be a blessing to me. Moments that I have felt a little sad or discouraged, his perspective and words of gratitude and surrender to the Lord bolstered my spirits.

What God is doing in and through him is truly amazing! I saw signs of it in so many of the staff, therapist, and other patients at rehab. They wanted to keep him until October! Too bad!

August 15, 2014

I told Brian he has become one of those people with the complicated medication regime! Lord Jesus, I hope this isn't forever. I have called the nurses' station four times and been to Walmart twice, and I have to

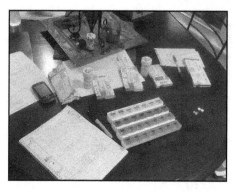

go to another pharmacy tomorrow because Walmart was out of one of the medications. Oh well, we are thankful for the meds and thankful he's here!

All the medications were overwhelming to me! However, Brian's mom and a visiting cousin helped me. I was too tired for their visit last night, but of course it ended up being a blessing. We got it all straight after a couple more calls to the nursing station at rehab... eight medications, spread out over four administration times through the day. I started a notebook and will get a four-section pill box. However, again another blessing—all the medications were free! So somewhere in the system Medicaid is being processed or we have met the deductible on insurance... either way, it's another sign that the Lord is my Provider!

Neither of us got much sleep last night. (Brian has a daybed set up in the living room since our only bathroom is on that level. I slept in our bed upstairs.) **But** he walked by himself from the living room to the bathroom with his cane unassisted five times between 11:00 PM and 8:30 AM so that is great!

This morning I admit I was feeling kind of discouraged. When your husband can't do some simple things like pour a glass of milk or dress himself, it is sobering. He needed help opening a water bottle, and I found myself tearing up. Then we heard the song "Garden" by NEEDTOBREATHE, and we both started crying. It was one we had often played together in worship. The refrain says, "Father, let my heart be after you." We looked at each other and wept. I said, "I want to hear you play this song." He said, "I don't care about playing it. I want to live it."

"Father, let my heart be after you." I so love that man. We were supposed to preach on husband-wife roles and submission at FWF July 13. The Lord is giving us an opportunity to learn by experience and walk it out. Also, it's a chance for me to follow my husband's lead once again.

I prayed the "Line Up Prayer" and asked for Jesus' strength... and to help me adopt Brian's perspective of being open to the process. *(Lord, as an act of my will, I surrender my spirit to Your Holy Spirit. I declare that my soul—my mind, will, and emotions—must be surrendered to my spirit, which is surrendered to Your Holy Spirit. I further declare that my body must line up and be surrendered under Your perfect authority. I ask this in Jesus' name.)*

After that he walked out to the studio for the first time, and we just had a good time enjoying each other.

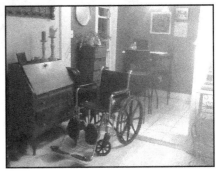

Not normal ... a wheelchair in the dining room. He hasn't used it yet though, probably won't unless we need to walk around a lot somewhere. Thankful to have it available though.

We did use it on one doctor appointment and got hysterical! I was pushing him through a slightly uphill parking lot... for those of you who don't know us, he's the size of a big football linebacker and I am ... not! So I accidentally spun it out, almost flipped him and nearly got him hit by a car!! Laughter is good medicine! (Proverbs 17:22 NLT)

August 15, 2014

Some semblance of normal ... guys watching a movie. Not so normal ... a daybed and cane in the living room. But that's okay. At least he's home!

I am trying to focus on being grateful and thankful! Brian and I both

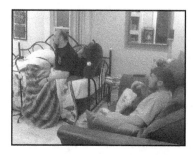

discussed that it is a little bittersweet coming home—because he can't do everything he is used to doing **yet**. We continue to pray and trust God in this **process**.

I think of people in the Bible who had to go through long processes to fulfill what God was calling them to do...Joseph, Moses, Job, the list is long. What about Zechariah (John the Baptist's father) whom God struck mute for nine months until his son was born? I continue to be amazed that anything we need and anything we are struggling with, there is wisdom and comfort and instruction in the Word. *"The Word is God is living and active, sharper than any double edged sword...." Hebrews 4:12 NIV*

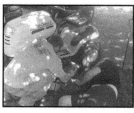 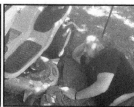

Mower issues. The neighbors mowed for me last week and will be glad to again, but we are trying to determine what's wrong so I can go get a new part. Brian walked outside with his cane, sat in a chair, but then got down on the ground to look underneath. He said it's hard to turn a ratchet wrench one handed, but he did it! It's so good to see Brian and Colton working on something! To this day he gives me tons of grief for "making him" go out there!

Brian: Adjusting to being home.
When I actually got home, it was quite an adjustment. After a day or two, after I just kind of rested and enjoyed being in my own place...then it sinks in... "Okay, I'm home, but I can't weed whack, paint the building, mow the grass, work in the garage or anything!" That's when I really started to realize how God provided friends who mowed the lawn, built ramps, installed railings on the stairs, and really, whatever else we needed.

The first time I sat on our beautiful wraparound deck again, I started to get a little inkling of resting in the Lord, a little tiny inkling. Okay, my strength is gone. I can't get up and do ___, I can't go to work. It's everything I can do to walk to the restroom or walk to the studio to read the Bible. However, God started to give me peace— "Just let it go. Just focus on Me. Don't worry about the Ferraris, your boss, getting the car done, playing the concert, the marriage sermon at church...don't worry about it." God was letting me focus on Him and Him alone.

I had no idea how long that time was going to be...I was thinking weeks, not years. I didn't know how long it was going to take me to unravel all the things in my life I had built up instead of God. It took me almost two years until I learned peace and freedom in Christ and what that really means—what His death on the cross did for us, for me—it took me two years for Him to show me that. But I got the first glimpse of it sitting on my deck that day with the sun beating down on me after being in the hospital five weeks, having my wife bring me a sandwich and glass of sweet tea.

Now that I've experienced that rest...I realize it comes from within, through the Holy Spirit. It doesn't have to do with our circumstances. It has to do with Christ. We can experience that rest absolutely anywhere. We might be in the busiest of times and we can still have inner tranquility. It doesn't matter what's happening around us. Our eternal promises with Him are sealed. We have a promise and an eternal hope...in what's coming!

I'm not saying I don't get frustrated, mad, or discouraged! I'm still human...but in those times I try to remind myself exactly what we have in Christ. As I catch myself, I can let the frustrations and the anger go. I only need to seek Him. He will fight the battle, take care of the details, make it all work out. I need to seek Him in all things, pray, and then do what I feel He's telling me to do—which is never to get angry and mad and throw a fit.

August 18, 2014

We planned a trip to Ohio with a missionary friend. Brian said, "It would be nice if the Lord would give me my hand back by then, so I could play. But it's God's timing."

Had a great walk this morning while I prayed the whole time. The Lord reminded me of a prophetic word Bri had received a few months before the stroke about "the cap" being removed... the limits being removed of where God wanted to take him. God tied it in with his feeling that he still has a bit of a "hat" on with the stroke. The Lord had me pray over him and break that off in Jesus' name.

August 19, 2014

I finished teaching piano lessons at 8:10 PM, and although I really didn't want to do it I dragged myself to the grocery store. Caught up with my mother on the phone and then ran into two dear folks in the dairy aisle. Stood for a long time catching them up on the stories of what God's been up to... every time I rehearse the praises it bolsters my spirits, which were a bit floppy today. When I got to the checkout line, the girl said, "Are you Sheila?" I nodded. She handed me a $100 bill. Said someone had left it to pay for my groceries.

I left feeling much lighter than when I had arrived. The Lord is so great at encouraging, and He enjoys using us in the process.

August 20, 2014

I had a little meltdown this morning. Sometimes the tears just come. Brian and I just held each other and cried. The song "Turn Your Eyes Upon Jesus" (written by Helen Howarth Lemmel) was playing on Pandora. He said, "Just listen to those words."

Yep. That's the secret.

August 21, 2014

Brian has been home one week. We are making adjustments... God has truly provided everything we need and we are grateful! I will be honest and say that I am weary—his needs, Garrett's needs, household needs, teaching—**but** I am sleeping well, and we have had some wonderful times together studying the Word, praying, talking, crying, just being.

Thank you for your prayers and support! Many people have asked what they can do. I don't know quite what to say. We have all the exercise equipment we need now. We have the carpet. The neighbor mowed the grass twice as our mower is waiting on a new belt.

Here are a couple things....

Aimee Patrick started a meal train for us. There is an online link or you can contact her.

My flower beds really need attention with weeding and our back patio has weeds growing up so badly it looks like a jungle! I am hoping to get some time tomorrow to be outside doing it. We'll see.

Today Bri has physical therapy in Woodstock and then a follow up with his doctor in Winchester. Hopefully afterwards we will get to enjoy dinner together at Olive Garden!

REALITY BEGINS TO SINK IN

*** *Looking back, I remember that during this time the reality of the situation was sinking in to me. It was a marathon, not a sprint! I do recall a sweet friend showing up soon after that previous post to weed my backyard. Sometimes when people would ask what they could do, I just wanted to say in a sharp, aggravated tone, "You can't do anything! Because the only thing I really want is for my husband to be totally normal again!"*

There were many, many occasions when I was so tired—physically, emotionally, and spiritually—of taking care of Brian and Garrett, all the house duties and the doctors, the piano students and ... and ... and.... Certainly, we all feel like that at times whether or not you've been through a stroke.

So what do we do? There are some practical things—such as eating healthy foods, getting some sleep even if that means lying down for a nap when you have tons to do! We can also spend time with people we know will bolster our spirits and encourage our faith. We can read the Bible even when we feel we're just staring at the words. We can listen to praise music even when we don't want to. We can let ourselves cry, allow ourselves to feel the grief, express the pain ... And then lay it before the Lord.

It's also important when going through a long-term care-giving process to occasionally do some things that completely remove you from the situation. Perhaps go out to lunch with a friend and talk about something different. Go window-shopping or do a creative project that stimulates the brain and the emotions. Exercise! Get those endorphins flowing. And realize that regardless of what this life holds, we truly are just pilgrims here. We are only passing through.

These are some of the things that were meaningful and helpful to me at that time.

August 24, 2014

Prayer request: sound, uninterrupted sleep! Both of us wake up multiple times per night for various reasons. I remember once when he was in the hospital I slept 6 hours straight. That felt so good!

August 25, 2014

We were given a sermon on CD with a central question: "What if the purpose of God is to teach you to see the joy of Who He is in the midst of your situation?" Wow.

Here's another question: "What does God want to be to me in this circumstance that He was unable to be any other time?" He wants to reveal a new facet of His nature or take me deeper than I have been before. That has been ringing in my mind and heart.

What were my answers today?... A loving servant, patience, joy, peace.

We received notice that our application for financial aid was approved by Valley Health (ER 7/10/14 and month in Winchester Rehab). They are covering us 100 percent! Praise God!! We are still waiting to hear about financial app for INOVA, Medicaid, and disability. We are trusting and know that He is our Provider.

I do request prayer for wisdom in some financial decisions we need to make. I have already repented because I realize part of my struggle is fear. And when fear is the root of something, it is never from God. But I do request wisdom and strength for obedience.

Brian has begun rehab therapy in Woodstock (10 minutes from home). He continues to make great progress and gains strength each day.

We are so very grateful! We were given several pieces of exercise equipment, and we turned one bay of the garage into a workout area. He has been out there a few times already. He continues to have such an inspirational God-focused attitude. While he completely believes the Lord could heal him instantly, he senses that God is saying, "Wait. The timing is not yet." This is a process, and we know the Lord has things to teach us in it and through it.

August 26, 2014

This morning while I drove Garrett to work at a sheltered workshop in town, Brian got his socks and shoes (including leg brace) on all by himself and walked from the house to the studio unassisted! Wow! That is a big deal!! Thank you, Lord!

August 27, 2014

Good news today! At therapy, they had Brian walking even without a cane! He was shaky, but he did it! Praise God! I couldn't go today because I was teaching, but I'm hoping to catch some video Friday. We continue to stand in awe of how the Lord is working in this situation.

Please continue to pray that both of us would **sleep** well. He has a sleep study scheduled for Sunday night. The neurologist in Fairfax thought sleep apnea was likely the underlying cause of the stroke, which is apparently a very common occurrence!

August 28, 2014

We both slept better last night! Thank you for the prayers! Keep them coming. I got out for a while today, just did some errands and such on my own. It was nice to just have some fun and get to clear my head. I had a couple gift cards too, so had some treats along the way. Brian enjoyed some time with "the guys" while I was gone, and I think that refreshed his spirit as well. He informed me that he made his own turkey sandwich for lunch … a difficult task when you do it with only one hand. Looking forward to Bible study tonight and more fellowship with friends.

August 30, 2014

Some notes from my Bible study yesterday down by the river. 1 Peter 2:21–24 (NIV)

"To this you were called, because Christ suffered for you, leaving you an example, that you should follow in his steps. He committed no sin, and no deceit was found in his mouth."

(Of course not, because Jesus **is** the Truth!)

"When they hurled their insults at him, he did not retaliate; when he suffered, he made no threats. Instead, he entrusted himself to him who judges justly."

This made me think of Job in the Bible launching into all the arguments, justifications, demands for explanations, questions and dialogue—trying to figure it all out when he was going through his horrendous trials … like we so often do as well when we suffer. Job's story ends with chapters 38–42 when God finally speaks and answers him. Job is struck with perspective and the reality of Who God is, which leads him right back into worship. Yep.

Then I went to Hebrews 5:7–9 NIV, *"During the days of Jesus' life on earth, he offered up prayers and petitions with loud cries and tears to the One who could save him from death, and he was heard because of his reverent submission."* So Jesus suffered! He felt the anguish and the frustration of his calling, of God's purpose. He cried out to the Father in that. **But** he was reverent in submission. Jesus chose to align himself with what God was doing and didn't even exert his own will for escape, which he could have done. See Luke 22:42 and Matthew 27:53–54.

Hebrews 5:10 NIV says, *"Son though he was, he learned obedience from what he suffered."*

Jesus was the Son of God; He was in fact, God (Colossians 2:9; Hebrews 1:3) Yet Jesus had things to learn through suffering. And if suffering was a good, God-appointed method to teach Jesus, how can I expect any less at some points in my life? And the key was that Jesus chose to align himself with the Father's purpose: He chose to submit to God's plan and to the circumstances in His life. If Jesus is my example, then that is my challenge as well.

And what did Jesus' submission lead to?

Hebrews 6:9 NIV: *"And, once made perfect, he became the source of eternal salvation for all who obey him."*

Back to 1 Peter 2:24 NIV: *"He himself bore our sins in his body on the cross, so that we might die to sin and live for righteousness; by his wounds you have been healed."*

Look at that good news! He took **my** sin. He paid the price. Why? Look at the invitation! **So that** I might die to sin and live to righteousness. WOW. *"By His wounds you have been healed."*

Brian: Reflections on acceptance

I can remember the first time I was able to ride the mower to cut grass. I thought, "At least I can do this." It felt good to do something normal, useful. I used to hate to cut grass. That day I realized how nice it was to be outside, to be warm, to cut the grass, wave at the neighbors. I remember that feeling. I still had to use the cane to walk to the mower—the four-prong cane, the "golden ticket" as we joked about it.

That cane got me preferential treatment all over the place. Lol. I think my friend Dusty was the first one to come and take me to lunch. I realized when you walk in with the four-prong cane, you automatically get a seat right by the door, right by the servers.

They put you at a table right away. They treat you a little differently. It opens doors and parts crowds.

I started to realize, "Hey, nothing is going to change the situation, so I might as well relax and make the best of it. Getting grumpy and thinking how much it stinks isn't going to make it better. It'll make it worse because you focus on negative." I began to enjoy that I could read or watch a show in the middle of the day, or take a nap. I didn't have to **do** anything, produce anything. And I started to get a little more glimpse of the **rest** and what God was wanting me to see. But I still was thinking, "Well, I'll do this for a time, but then I'll start doing stuff to get back to normal.

Later I realized, "No, it's the **normal** that God wants to heal me from!" He wants to make us extraordinary. And that is different in God's terms than the world...I Hear Him, talk to Him, Scripture comes alive when I read. The one living God, who created everything, put it into motion and holds it in motion is communicating with me! Not one sparrow falls from the sky without the Lord seeing it. Take heed: if He saved me in this flesh from death, He didn't save me so that I could sit in the living room watching endless episodes of *Rockford Files* on Netflix. He saved me for a purpose. I wanted to hear Him in that purpose, follow Him in that purpose.

Out of the stroke and therapy, God started to build a quiet resolve in me that I was not going to quit. I was going to obey. I was going to find out who I was in Him and find out what He wanted me to do.

September 1, 2014

Right now Bri is still sleeping on a daybed downstairs in our living room since there is no bathroom upstairs. But he decided today to climb the stairs for the first time and did great! Going up was really pretty easy he said. Coming down was more challenging, but he did it! Thanks again to friends from our church for the new sturdy railings!

Brian had his sleep study last night in Winchester. The tech was able to determine after a very short amount of time that he definitely has sleep apnea, a quite severe case. She hooked him up to a CPAP machine at 1:15 AM and he did not move or awaken at all until she woke him at almost 6:00 AM! He never does that! He woke feeling refreshed, rejuvenated, and he mentioned that his left arm and left leg felt better. Also, he said the feeling of the "warm towel" around the base of his neck that has been there since the stroke had lessened as well. We are grateful and look forward to getting the machine in a few days. With better oxygen levels to his brain as well as his whole body, we look forward to accelerated improvements. Thanks for your prayers!

September 3, 2014

> Check out 1 Peter 2:25 NIV, *"For you were like sheep going astray, but now you have returned to the Shepherd and Overseer of your souls."*

> And then Job 10:12 NIV, *"You gave me life and showed me kindness, and in your providence watched over my spirit."*

September 4, 2014

Update after Brian's PT (physical therapy) today ... please pray specifically for strength, movement, and flexibility in his knees and ankle. His knee still wants to do a "snapping" motion ... the muscles just need to be built up. He feels that his ankle is key for him to be able to walk better. He did walk along the hall in therapy barely holding on to the rail ... i.e.: no cane, no railing! Yeah!

Therapist did say that a stationary bike would be a good thing for him to have. We have an elliptical machine, which he has tried to do. The movement and balance required in that is just a little too much yet.

If someone has a stationary bike we can borrow ... thanks!

September 5, 2014

Please pray that Brian will get his CPAP machine today. I am making my kind but persistent phone calls. Lol. He couldn't sleep last night until 5:00 AM. We learned from Amy Gray, a new OT (occupational therapist) this week, how extremely crucial good sleep is for the healing process! Our bodies need it! God designed it that way and there are certain chemicals that are only released when we sleep which restore our systems. So....if your body is telling you to rest, then **rest**!

One of Brian's coworkers just stopped by to say hi. There is a man in the community who sometimes stops by their shop. He had commented to the guys, "Did that one guy quit?" They explained what had happened to Brian. The man stopped back around the shop today with a check in hand. It's for $500 from a men's group at a local church, people we don't even know. Wow. God is just so gracious!

September 8, 2014

OT homework is interesting! Therapist said anything he can do standing up engages his brain more. This exercise is moving bottles from one quadrant to the opposite one, because our brains operate in quadrants. Crossing those quadrants of the brain gets it fired up!

Please continue to pray for our strength for the long haul to recovery. **But** we focus on Jesus and are **so** grateful for day-by-day progress!

*** *And looking back, that truly had to be my emphasis in order to survive: focusing on Jesus and counting our blessings every day. It was an incredibly difficult time. Yet we experienced amazing and frequent blessings.*

Notes from my journal during my quiet time today:

This recovery for Brian is a slow process. Although there is much that he now can do, there is still much he cannot do. Lord, give us strength, patience, perseverance for the long haul.

I ask again, "Lord, what do you want to do to me in this time?" and

I get the sense that He wants to show me how He is the God of all time. That there is no sense of urgency with Him, no deadlines, because His timing is perfect. After all, He created time to begin with! All times are in His hands; all time is His season, and to Him a day is like a thousand years. Lord, I thank you and praise you for Who you are, Great God of time and infinite in power, presence, and wonder!

And I stand on the promise You gave me at the beginning of this journey—that Brian will be totally healed and totally whole. (Yes, I sensed the Holy Spirit speaking that to my heart in the first moments of the stroke.) When I moaned about it 48 hours in, the Lord said, "I told you he will be fine. What difference does it make how long it takes?"

Help me, Lord. Give me more faith. Open my eyes to see your perspective. Open my lips to praise you in the midst of the journey. Let us lay down what our flesh wants and walk in what Your Spirit is doing. In Jesus' name, Amen.

September 9, 2014

Just got the word from my sweet friend/secretary Aimee Patrick that she spoke to INOVA this morning saying we had never heard back about our financial aid app. The lady said, "Well, your balance on everything is zero!" Apparently, Anthem paid and INOVA accepted that as payment in full. **Thank You, Lord**! Separate doctors might bill us, but we will handle that as it comes.

Still waiting on CPAP machine and trusting God's perfect timing.

Brian would like specific prayer for his left knee: although he is walking fairly easily, his left knee still "snaps/locks" in place. He is sensing that the Lord is using this physical issue to speak to him some spiritual truths as well. So just lift that up, please. Thanks.

We got the stationary bike today from Brian's uncle, and are getting the Bowflex machine this week also, both of which will help strengthen hamstring muscles too.

Of course, of even greater concern to him is that he would be able to play guitar again. He misses it! But he knows that it's in God's hands and trusts His timing.

September 10, 2014

CPAP machine pick up and consultation scheduled for Monday, September 15, in Woodstock. That was the soonest they could do, but she will call me if there are any cancellations sooner. Poor guy needs sleep, although **thank you** for praying because both of us have slept better this last week.

THE CONTINUING PROCESS OF RECOVERY

Brian: on walking

You mentioned about the left leg and that the Lord wanted to teach me something through that. I can't say that I know exactly what He was trying to say, but I know that one of the things was about our walk. I've found that one of the things with the stroke is I couldn't look around when I was walking. I had to stay focused on where I was going and where I was stepping. And that's a very spiritual parallel! We have to be focused on where we're going.

Paul admonished believers to keep their *"eyes on the prize, as one trying to gain the prize."* (Philippians 3:14; 1 Corinthians 9:24–27 NIV) We are to be focused on Christ, and we always have to watch where we're putting our feet—Is it on something firm? If I would step on a rock or a little hole in the ground, it would almost make me fall because my left foot, leg, and ankle couldn't compensate for the change in terrain. I had to be on fairly level ground or I was wobbly. I think there's a spiritual symbolism to that: we need to seek out level ground to walk on. Otherwise we easily are thrown off balance. We can't be looking around at everything—distractions! The world wants to show us the latest shiny thing, but that is not what helps us focus on Christ. If something doesn't help us to center on Christ, then it leads us away from Christ which is onto—we know who. There is no other option.

You're either focusing on Christ Jesus or you're focusing on Satan. Because when you're absorbed with yourself or your own needs, you're not really trusting Jesus. When you're focused on the world, you're not focused on Christ. God knows your needs; He knows your wants and desires. He knows when emergencies arise in your life. He sees all the drama. We don't need to dwell on it. We just need to be riveted on Him and He will solve the problems in the way He sees fit. And I guarantee that the way He irons out the problems is better in the long run than the way I would solve them.

September 10, 2014 Facebook post:

OT today ... so interesting! Did you know that the progress on the left leg is key for the improvement of the left arm? So walking is the best exercise he can do, which helps overall. The emphasis at this point is fine motor skills which are the last thing to come back. I am praying for "lightning speed in the name of Jesus!" However, actually my prayer since the beginning of this journey (nine weeks tomorrow) is, "Lord, I pray that you would have mercy and shorten this process as much as possible which would still allow for everything You wish to accomplish."

Same day ... a private email to a close friend:

I am okay. Feeling a little "stuck" in the recovery journey. **But** must focus on the positive and all the things that he has improved in. We got word yesterday from INOVA that all of our bills are zero balance, so **praise** GOD!

We are both struggling with how this changes our plans for moving to Texas. But that's just what God is confirming—they were **our** plans. The stroke and this process were never surprises to the Lord. He knew all along. I found in my prayer walk yesterday that I had to lay down my own expectations, timing, plans, and repent for the fear, pride, and selfishness involved. Brian has a stiff knee (it wants to lock and snap instead of bending and moving smoothly), and yesterday my neck and shoulders were stiff. We contemplated possible spiritual parallels. What God revealed is that perhaps those physical issues are signs of a heart attitude with both of us, and have prayed about that. I think we need to pray together about it and go to God together, but I tend to "push" him with that kind of stuff which frustrates him. I need to just wait.

I'm struggling to just rest and be calm in the moment and not plan and purpose for next steps whether it be recovery or life plans. I prayed yesterday, "Lord, my brain just can't figure all this out… good thing it's not up to my brain then, huh?!"

September 14, 2014
Brian: Then
At this point in the recovery, I think I was starting to struggle with not getting angry and not getting impatient with people. Because so many people—my wife included—were in some ways looking at me thinking, "Well, come on, get over this. Get back to normal. Pick that up. Do this with your left side. Just do it!" And of course I just couldn't. As hard as I tried, my left hand, foot, ankle, shoulder just wouldn't do what I wanted them to do. It's as if your body has forgotten. It just won't move the way you want it to. You can't hold things; you can't grip. Just flipping a light switch was a challenge.

Sheila, as loving as she was, was trying to get me to do things around the house. She figured as long as I was around all the time, I might as well help her with some chores. And I just couldn't. So I think I was starting to show some frustration at myself and at others. Then I realized the Lord was trying to show me something through these instances. You know we jokingly say, "You don't want to pray for patience!" But God is teaching me patience through this recovery. This is the hardest thing I have ever had to do. I've never really been sick or hurt where I couldn't just bounce back quickly and go back to normal, to play with pain so to speak.

I can't do that with this. The funny thing (true blessing!) is that I'm not—never have been through the whole stroke process —been in any pain. It doesn't hurt. My left side just won't work the way I want it to work. Physically, as far as health is concerned, I've actually felt the best I have in years!

Back at that time, I just couldn't move the way I wanted to move. I couldn't pick things up. I couldn't run, walk, or jump the way I always had. Through it all, including the financial challenges, the Lord showed me that He had never left my side! He was continuing in ways—that I didn't even see until they were completed—to provide for us, to help, to see us through.

Many people watching us through the whole process wondered, "How do you not have to declare bankruptcy?" A little later in the story we'll share our experience with the credit cards. When the money did finally start to dwindle, there were a couple things the Lord really wanted to teach us financially. It's amazing what He showed me in that! Through it all, we weren't missing payments. Our electric bill was current. Our mortgage was current. There was food in our cupboards. We had gasoline to get around. There was even some money for some extra things once in a while. My wife and I could get away and go out to eat occasionally, or to take the kids out for pizza. It wasn't like we were just sitting at home eating cans of tuna or something. He never left us destitute.

***And see, the Lord told me that at the beginning. That was something I sensed very early on ... "You will not be made poor in this situation or through it. It will really not affect you negatively financially." I also had this experience more than once: people (especially women) looking me in the eye and saying, "How are you doing this? How are you surviving?" I would answer, "By the strength and grace of God." That sounds like a trite religious mantra; however, I had never meant it more in my entire life! All those verses of Scripture that proclaim God is our strength, our fortress in trouble, our provider, our comforter ... those are "not just idle* *words for you. They are your life." (Deuteronomy 32:47 NIV) Yep. Lived it. As my mother said recently facing a potentially bad medical report, "We either believe God or we don't. It's really that simple. And if we do believe Him, then we know He will take care of us regardless of the circumstances."*

September 14, 2014 Another private email to a close friend:
I am wrestling and vacillating between wanting (and needing) to have a servant's heart versus really wanting to pamper myself, do what I want to do or feel I need. It is **not** wrong to care for ourselves. Particularly in the midst of a long haul trauma and life change, we need times of refreshment emotionally, physically, and spiritually. Think of the rule on airplanes: "In the event of an emergency or loss of cabin pressure, the oxygen masks will descend. If you are traveling with small children, put your own mask on first and then assist others." That goes against every bone in a normal mother's body. And yet if I don't take care of myself, how will I be able to take care of anyone else?

Growing up, I had watched my mother put everyone's needs ahead of her own most of the time. Especially in later years caring for my father (seventeen years older than she) and also my brother who has Down's syndrome. I truly saw her as a loving, nurturing servant…and quite frankly, I am not happy about walking in those same footsteps. My flesh is screaming out about it.

I had grown accustomed to my three men clearing out in the mornings, leaving me to the whole day at home. Yes, plenty of chores taking care of a household and teaching part time, but plenty of time alone for quiet reflection, investing in hobbies and relationships, as well as intimacy with the Lord. With the drastic change of our lifestyle and the demands falling on me, I am struggling. It is what it is. This is what is required of me right now. So I pray a lot, rest when I can, steal moments of nurturing for myself when and where I can, and just keep going.

I remember one day particularly that I was whining to God about feeling like a servant. I said, "I don't want to be a servant!" He said, "Jesus was a servant. So you don't want to be like Jesus?" Ouch. Repentance and prayer followed for a changed perspective.

Although it is not wrong to take care of ourselves and at times even put our own needs first, that still must be directed by God. Even Jesus went away by himself at times; He took care of himself. He knew what would refresh his spirit. This is another opportunity to crucify my flesh and be unselfish. At times, when I have examined my thoughts and listened to my tone in my responses, I could easily see my "flesh." What/how I was saying was not what Jesus would have said/done. God is teaching me a lot.

I do appreciate prayers as I wrestle this out with the Lord. Thank you.

*** *As time went on, I understood more about the challenges caretakers face. It changes ones perspective of his/her spouse to see them in a weakened state, depending on your help and support. As a wife, I think it's easy to then begin to view your husband as a child rather than a strong, independent man. It changes the relationship—emotionally, physically, sexually. And it's easy for the caregiver to lose his/her identity because every ounce of energy gets consumed by the other's needs. Perhaps codependency could occur as well.*

*Now at this writing—three-plus years after the stroke—because Brian has recovered so well, I find it is time to switch gears back to a more normal relationship. I do not need to continue doing so much for him! That is a little bit challenging to stop doing just as it was challenging to start doing! Right now, he is in Virginia for a month preaching and teaching at FWF to give Bryan and Aimee a break. He flew across the country, changing planes in Dallas Fort Worth airport and managing his own medications as well as therapy, workouts, meals, and daily life. I believe this break is God-ordained as well, as we both discern it's time to adjust **out** of the caregiver/receiver role. Interesting.*

I wrote this note to include with the thank-you notes we sent to people and churches that had sent donations:

9/15/14 Brian's recovery…praise update…Brian was released from Rehab on 8/14/14 and was very glad to get home. He continues to make excellent progress and gains strength every day. We are exceedingly grateful that he lost **no** memories or cognitive function! Currently he is walking without assistance using a four-prong cane and is beginning to work in therapy on walking without one. His speech is almost completely normal! Left arm, wrist and hand have movement but just not much strength yet. He is working now on a lot of fine motor skills in occupational therapy, and the therapist is excellent! Please pray specifically for continued movement and strength in his left ankle, wrist and hand, particularly so he can play his guitar again. Also, pray that we would clearly hear the Lord's guidance for our next steps in ministry, work, etc. And please pray against discouragement and irritability for both of us. This is a marathon journey.

We heard that Valley Health (ER and one month Rehab) approved our financial aid app 100 percent! Praise the Lord! And INOVA (six days ICU plus one day regular) said our balance was zero. Anthem paid, and they apparently wrote off the rest. So the Lord took care of way over $100K worth of medical bills! There are still a few pending, but we know He will provide. Medicaid and Disability are pending. We discovered this week a rather major problem with our house foundation and water drainage that needs to be addressed. Thankfully, we know professionals in the field who are working on bids.

Although certainly this has been a difficult season, we know that the Lord has a good plan! One thing in particular that we have learned is to focus on **who** God is and asking Him who He wants to be to us during this time. He certainly has been Provider, generously meeting our needs financially and in every other way. **Thank you** so much for your gift. We have been blown away by His generosity through the Body of Christ! If you are on Facebook, send a message to us via "Sheila Lin Mooney Lloyd." We have set up a Facebook page with all of his updates and videos.

September 15, 2014

> My Bible study this morning was 1 Peter 3:15 NIV: *"In your*
> *hearts, set apart Christ as Lord … always be prepared to give*
> *an answer to everyone who asks you about the hope that*
> *you have…."*

It is no secret that this journey of recovery is a marathon rather than a sprint. Although Brian has made wonderful progress, the dailiness of it gets wearisome. **But** with that Scripture verse, I was convicted to list out some **praises**!

Brian is alive, home, and cognitively excellent! His speech is nearly normal. His personality is unaltered (except for the transformation which the Lord is working).

He can walk!

There are many things he can now do for himself that he struggled with even a couple weeks ago—getting a shower, putting on deodorant with his left hand, getting dressed (including socks, brace, and shoes).

Valley Health approved our financial aid app 100 percent. That covers ER and the month in Rehab.

INOVA says our bill balance is zero. Anthem paid, and they apparently wrote off the rest.

Food stamps are a blessing! Yep, had to swallow my pride, but this is the reason the system exists, and Brian has paid into it since he was fifteen.

Sleep study revealed what is probably the root issue of the high BP and stroke—sleep apnea. He is being fitted for his CPAP machine today. With proper sleep and increased oxygen going to his brain/body, we expect wonderful progress in healing. (Please, if you're reading this and struggle with feeling lethargic all the time or severe snoring, go get a CT and a sleep study!)

Brian has met our insurance deductible, so all of his meds (which are substantial—pray they are not forever) are no charge.

Friends and family have been **incredibly** supportive with **whatever** we need over these last ten weeks … money, meals, rides, things at the house, help with administrative stuff, shoulders to cry on, and **prayers**.

The boys are going through this storm just fine, praise Jesus!

We have an opportunity to get away a few days and visit one of the churches in Ohio that sent us support. We're looking forward to being ministered to as well as sharing testimony, and we are excited about what the Lord has in store.

I know I could continue on and on. **Thank you, Lord**! That is **a lot** to be thankful for.

Yes, continued prayer requested for healing, perseverance, and work that needs to be done to fix a water drainage problem and a section of our basement wall. We have friends who are professionals in the field working up quotes. Foundation issues on your home are a sobering thought, **but** God has been faithful … **and** He will continue to be! Because that is Who He is. It is His character.

Thank **You** for your support on this journey. **Give GOD the praise!**

September 15, 2014
Brian: Then and Now
That trip to Ohio was good I needed that trip for God to show me that I am not useless. I can do things. I can get out. The trip was not hard on me. I could travel, although I couldn't drive yet. God showed me that I could still minister. I could still talk about God and encourage people.

Garrett traveled along with us on that trip. That's when God started to give me the idea that Garrett is a part of whatever He wants to do. Garrett has a role to play in ministry. He ministers to people. A little while later I had the dream about G and I driving around in a green classic Ford 100 pickup truck. We were driving around the country ministering to people wherever we went. It was not actually formal ministry but just driving around, meeting people at the gas station or at cafes or whatever, and Garrett would just make connections with people. We'd end up praying with them or leading them to the Lord or showing them things that God was doing. It was amazing! He showed me everything so clearly. I can tell you what year the truck was—1977 F100, two-wheel drive, short bed, but it had a wood bed (as far as the floor with the wood strips, and that was odd because they don't normally have that). I know what kind of wheels it had. It was a five-speed, and I was physically fine—able to drive it. (At the time of the dream I couldn't do that, and even today—April 2017—I would have a hard time doing that proficiently.) In the dream I was physically just fine: I could get out, fix things that would go wrong, change a tire, help Garrett do things. I was in great shape.

That's one of the dreams that I've had, just one of them because there have been many. But that one was the beginning—where God is showing me that I'm fine in the dreams—running, jumping, physically in very good shape. I'm not sure what God is trying to tell me in that; I don't claim to be an interpreter of dreams. Those are just dreams I've had. Plenty of people have told me the green truck means ministry … all this stuff. I don't know. God will let me know when I need to know. However, what it did show me was that He is not done with me. The real picture is not just of my being close to fifty, having a health issue, and "Boom!" I'm done. No. I may be done with a certain part of my life, but I'm not finished. He's morphing me into something new, and it's better. I'm going to be better than I was before, both physically and spiritually.

Sheila: Yes, That's what He told me at the very beginning while the stroke was happening: You would be completely restored, better than new.

Brian: He's making me new. I've had to give up a lot that I thought was important. But I'm gaining things that God thinks are important. And I'm learning that that is much better! It's always much better. I have more peace. He's showing me more about peace in these last couple years than I ever knew was possible. I'm so thankful to Him for that.

September 18, 2014

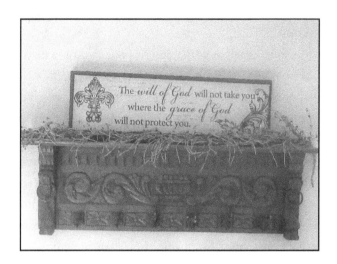

September 22, 2014

We returned last night from our trip to Ohio. We appreciated the fellowship and just enjoyed some rest and change of scenery. Garrett came along because the Lord has shown that he will often travel with us in the season of ministry that is coming. He did **great**!

It was interesting five days with CPAP machine, meds, and a Down's/autistic person in tow. But God gave strength, lessons, and much joy along the way.

We heard challenging messages in the fear of the Lord … see Isaiah 11:1–3. It says Jesus delighted in the fear of the Lord. I want to study and gain a fuller understanding of what that means. If Jesus delighted in it, why don't we? How can we?…

September 25, 2014

Just wanted to report a praise that both Brian and I are sleeping better!

He is getting used to his CPAP machine and now sleeping for 4 or more hours at a time and dreaming, which means he is getting some deep sleep. Oxygen to the brain and good sleep are key elements of healing.

I, too, have been sleeping for longer periods more soundly. Last night I slept over 6 hours straight! Haven't done that since he was in INOVA. Thank you, Lord!

I wrote this in an email to a friend in response to some things she was sharing in her own life … kind of sums things up well at this point:

I definitely understand about waking up in the "alternative" life and just wanting things to be back to "normal." And yet I remember Barbara Johnson at a Women of Faith conference years ago saying, "Normal is just a setting in your dryer." Also, like you, I don't think things will ever be exactly the same again because God is transforming us … through these refining fires, purifying, burning off what is left of our flesh and our desires and our expectations. And so I have to be honest and say I don't want to be like I was prior to all this. Also, the incredible beauty and faith I see in my husband is something I would not want to see go away (even though I often realize how anxious I am to just have him "back to normal" physically). Yes, through these challenges God is taking away our "props" like having a job to pay the bills, in order that we learn how to truly and fully rely on Him. Easier said than done. But He is so very faithful! We truly do not feel anxious. On paper the financials don't really make sense, and yet we are fine. All our bills are current.

*** *Looking back, I realized God had laid a foundation all along for us to endure this journey. Garrett's birth in 1997 and diagnosis of Down's syndrome (and six years later of Autism) provided similar opportunities to trust God and find joy on a marathon journey. The Bible says that God in His grace does not give us more than we can handle. Certainly, as humans we question His scales at times! But scripture says He moves us from "glory to glory" or "strength to strength." And He never ever ever leaves us or forsakes us. We truly can hold on to those promises regardless of what life brings. (See Psalm 84; Hebrews 13:5; Isaiah 42:16 NIV)*

September 25, 2014

At the recommendation of Brian's PT, we went to see a specialist who can custom make a brace (AFO) for his foot which has hinges that will allow more movement and flexibility in the toes and ankle as he continues to recover. I thought the lady's voice sounded familiar. When I saw her face I knew right away—she was the same person who made custom orthotics for Garrett when he was about four years old! Wow! Blast from the past. Bri with his usual sense of humor had her in stitches the whole time. Now just pray Anthem will pay for it!

September 30, 2014

Brian is asking for specific prayer: for his shoulders. He is in pain—he hasn't had pain through this whole thing. His right shoulder is sore because of the extra emphasis and compensation. His left shoulder is sore, therapists say, because of the stroke. The brain hasn't had to pay much attention to those nerves and now they are trying to move more, hence the pain.

Also, Anthem will only cover a certain number of therapies. He only has a couple more left. Medicaid and Disability are still pending. When those kick in, he can have many more appointments.

This is the stage of recovery that gets discouraging because most of the work now is fine motor skills, which take longer. He is getting bored, and yet the things that he loves to do he is not able to do yet. So pray for him please.

We are both weary of this process (almost twelve weeks) **but** we are trusting the Lord and trying to focus on Him, His plan, and His many blessings in the midst of it. Thank you for your prayers! We continue to believe for complete healing and restoration.

Brian's testimony recorded September 30, 2014:

Good morning (as he waves his left hand deliberately). I want to thank everybody for all their prayers and continuing to pray for me as God takes me on this journey. I know it's a journey where I'm learning about God's process of healing. Sure, I know God can heal me, does heal, and He can heal me instantly if He wants. But there is something I have to learn in this process. Part of that is patience and perseverance and just waiting. I keep thinking of Psalm 40, waiting patiently for the Lord. There's something in that I'm supposed to learn. We're waiting patiently for the Lord as I get better. He will make me better when He wants me to do something—when He's ready for me to move forward in the task He has before me. Not until then. Because if I get better before then, I won't appreciate it. I'll take it for granted. I need to learn the road of walking out this healing. Working for it. I appreciate everybody's prayers. I really do. I know He hears our prayers and answers them. I'm getting stronger every day. There's something new every day. Today my hand just feels really good. My arm is feeling better. My shoulder is feeling better; it's not hurting nearly as much. I thank everybody for their prayers and keep it up. Bye.

October 3, 2014
Bri was able to eat corn on the cob at dinner tonight … holding it in both hands. Yeah!

October 1, 2014 … (*** *Only one year later we left VA moving to Texas!*) Thanks for the prayers about the number of visits Brian has for therapy. He must have misunderstood. We were there today and cleared it up. He has appointments through the end of October. Hopefully by then we will have received a determination from Medicaid and/or Disability. The OT believes because of a stroke he will be approved the first time for Disability. Thanks for the continued prayers!

October 6, 2014
Brian had an appointment with our family doctor today. She as well as her nurse have been getting all the reports since the stroke, but this was the first time they saw him in person. They were both just ecstatic and

joining us in giving God the praise. They have been watching and reading the reports in amazement this whole time! Also, the doctor didn't think his course of meds was that much considering all he's been through. She also reviewed the fasting blood work he had taken last Thursday ... everything was extremely good she said. We are just **so grateful** to the Lord for all He's done and continuing to do.

We are still waiting on Medicaid and/Disability, so you can be in prayer about that please.

Also, his shoulders still get quite sore. Sleeping is going much better for both of us! Yeah!

October 7, 2014 Brian: deeply moved by a friend's visit...
We had a visit with our friend. He just wanted to come over to give us a gift of several household items that he and his wife had

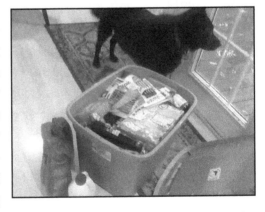

been saving up to bless us. And it was a blessing! But also, I think he just wanted to tell us how God was using our situation in his life. It was humbling. In the early stages of the stroke journey, I was kind of irritated that Sheila was putting my whole life on Facebook. I felt like I was starring in a reality show. But then our friend shared with us what his family had gone through and how God had used my testimony. As he watched God bringing me through this hard thing, he was able to gain encouragement and strength to persevere in his own struggle.

When you hear that, for me anyway, it was just like, "Wow, God, I'm not worthy. I'm just a guy who's struggling with how to cope with what has happened. But one way you were allowing me to cope, Lord, was in helping someone else. So if that's the case, if it helps someone else, then who am I to say that this is too hard or that this is too much? I'll endure what you want me to endure to reach who you want me to reach if that's the case."

That was just one of those moments when you realize that it's not just about me! There's a whole world of people who need to be reached and encouraged for the Lord Jesus. Even if they are believers, they need to be encouraged and strengthened because we all go through stuff. We need to minister to one another. We need to be there for one another, to listen and share what God brings us. We all are uniquely equipped to help someone else. (See 2 Corinthians 1:3–11; 1 Thessalonians 5:11)

I'm thankful that I was able to provide encouragement for a friend, a good friend.

October 7, 2014

Well, I had a checkup at our family doctor yesterday and was absolutely shocked at my weight. She was not at all concerned about it...said the scale always ran heavy. She's middle-aged and was actually kind of funny talking about the hot flashes, purging old clothes sizes, etc. But it was a wake-up call for me. I am not comfortable in my own skin, and the image in the mirror just doesn't look like me. I had a good long journaling session with the Lord last night and came to some good conclusions...lots of the spiritual sides to this issue (God loves me regardless, accepting myself, etc.) but also my conclusions including that it is time for me to change some things.

Besides my frustrations with my weight and premenopausal issues (such great fun being a woman!), I have had some moments the last couple days of just being tired of this journey, just wanting my husband back. But I'm okay.

It was a good day. I had some good time of bible study, got to work on a stained glass, and then this evening had a visit from a friend. He sat and shared about some really difficult things they have been going through in their family since May and how the Lord has used our testimonies on the Facebook page to encourage his faith. We were fairly blown away. Tonight Brian said, "Yep, give me another stroke if that's the benefit." Wow.

October 8, 2014 OT today:
Imprinting into putty. It gives about a pound of resistance. It's working this index finger that will be very useful for playing guitar again. Keep praying. We are believing for total healing and restoration in Jesus' name!

October 10, 2014 Facebook post
There are certainly times lately when we look at each other and say, "Are we done with this yet?" The process gets wearisome. However, we got a great word of encouragement from a physical therapist today, "Looking back it seems like a long time, but looking forward it's just a small amount of time. Next year at this time this will just be a small chunk. You are way back in the game!" Thank you, Lord, for that.

October 10, 2014 PRIVATE JOURNAL
This morning I just felt blue, frustrated, irritated, and wanting to be left alone. I reflected on 2014 for me…decision to move across country, parents' declining health, and choices that go along with that, Brian suffering the stroke July 10, Dad's death August 2, Brian coming home August 15 but needing quite a bit of care and support, therapy and doctor appointments, long-term marathon recovery, premenopausal and all the fun stuff that goes along with that (weight gain and hot flashes!), and going from lots of time alone to 24/7 pretty much with hubby who has TV or music on almost all the time, often even through the night. I guess looking at all of that, my feelings make sense. Lol.

But I realize that it is not about me. It's about God. So in my quiet time this morning (when I could finally get out to the studio), I sank into my chair and just caught one verse I had written in my notebook yesterday, *"Cast all your cares on Him because He cares for you."* (1 Peter 5:7

NIV) Through a little cry fest, I physically handed over all the stressors to the Lord.

That is where I am today.

*** *And that entry perfectly describes why journaling is valuable! In this fast-paced world where we are bombarded with millions of forms of stimulation every day—perhaps every hour—we need to be able to get quiet and take stock in our life. Our emotions, which run rampant and cause significant stress, difficulty, conflict, and eventually even physical ailments, need to be evaluated and recognized so they can be processed in a healthy manner.*

Thoughts About Worship

October 11, 2014

Brian and I read an article about Sunday morning worship music. Here are his comments... I had to type fast!

Sunday morning is not meant to be how we get our faith or how to get our Christianity. It's meant to be a celebration of what God has done throughout the week in our lives.

Also, read about the kingdom of David... everyone else had two to three jobs, but the musicians' only job was playing music. Their job was night and day. Music was playing 24/7 in David's reign, and they were never invaded. It proclaims God's presence, His power, His glory. And when God is glorified and honored, the enemy must flee. Where two or more are gathered, God is there.

We should worship; music is part of that. But it doesn't have any magical powers. However, when we are gathered corporately in agreement in worship, that is powerful! Why do you think the musicians went ahead of the soldiers into the battle? Because it was proclaiming God. It was His power that was winning the battle, and the music proclaimed that. (2 Chronicles 20)

Don't underestimate the power of music in worship. It's part of God's plan. Music is emotional. It moves us emotionally. It cuts through barriers and breaks down walls (emotional and real). Look at Paul and Silas ... the walls of the jail were broken down. It wasn't the music. It was God's power. (See Acts 16)

Who was Lucifer? He was the angel of worship. In fact, he actually embodied all the instruments (Isaiah 14), and he has tried to pervert music. Music was meant to glorify God, not us! But too many people worship worship but do not worship God. Music does get you in the emotional state where you are receptive to God's word. Music should prepare our hearts to hear God, so then the one who is proclaiming the Word has a receptive audience—that is the job of the worship leader. The people are ready to listen because they have gotten rid of their other junk. They are now at the point where they are worshipping God and ready to receive.

Music is never meant to displace God's word but reinforce it. Sunday morning service is about proclaiming God's power. Worship is one of the main ways we do that, and we do it with music. Because then everyone can worship and come before God in unity.

Okay, wow! Great thoughts. I wholeheartedly agree. Guess that's why we are worship leaders!

October 12, 2014

Today leading worship I was frustrated because we are having issues with some white noise feedback in our sound system when my keyboard is on. It was buzzing in my ear the entire time. However, the Lord used it as an object lesson for me—the world will constantly try to distract us from focusing on Jesus. We have a choice whether to give in to the distraction or to strive even harder to focus more on Him. This realization came while we were singing the song *"Turn your eyes upon Jesus. Look full in His wonderful face. And the things of earth will grow strangely dim in the light of His glory and grace."* I so appreciate how the Lord teaches me!

SMALL STEPS

October 13, 2014

Praise Report…Brian just walked into the kitchen (without a cane—which he has been doing the past week or more around the house) and said, "Well, I think my foot is finally starting to act like a foot!" The explanation…he got a new custom cast orthotic Thursday afternoon for his left foot. (Handmade by Sarah at Valley Orthotics, the same woman who made them for Garrett when he was little.) This brace, unlike the ones in the past, allows a lot more natural movement for his foot and ankle, while holding his foot and leg in a better position. One big thing is that it lets him step onto his heel first rather than the ball of his foot. He says another benefit of the brace is that his knee is feeling stronger. **Yeah**! Go, God! Thank you for praying! Keep it up!

October 18, 2014

Today Brian is helping his former OT from Rehab fix the brakes on his car. Not sure if he is turning the wrenches or just directing someone else to turn them, but regardless he is getting stronger! Pretty cool that this was the first therapist who evaluated him when he was admitted there 7/18/14 and couldn't hardly move his left arm or leg!

I dropped him off and visited our sweet neighbor who was admitted to hospice Thursday night. She is a delightful woman, and it was a blessing to be able to visit with her, talk with her about the Lord, and tell her how much I have enjoyed her. Also at hospice, I stopped in to visit Pamela, a woman we met on the patio a couple days before Brian came home. (Rehab is floor 3; hospice is floor 4.)

October 19, 2014
Brian and I finally made it up to Skyline Drive Friday! It was a gorgeous day, perfect temp and breathtaking views.

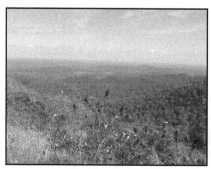 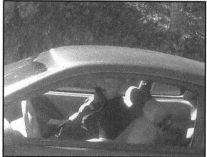

October 21, 2014
Yesterday, Brian was blessed by a therapeutic massage from a friend.. Wow! What difference it made to his pain level and also his range of motion! We are very grateful!

October 22, 2014
Some recent Bible study notes

> 1Peter 5:9 NIV: *"Resist him (the devil who is prowling around), standing firm in the faith...."*

I did a word study on standing firm a while back which was extremely interesting. Right now the "standing firm" verse that jumps out at me is Ephesians 6:13 NIV: *"Therefore (since our struggle is not against flesh and blood but spiritual forces), put on the full armor of God, so that when the day of evil comes you will be able to stand your ground, and after you have done everything, to stand."*

My NIV Study Bible text note says the imagery there in the Greek is not of a massive invasion, but of individual soldiers withstanding assault. Lord Jesus, I ask for your renewed strength upon us and within us during this season of Brian's recovery. Some days we grow weary and discouraged. **But** we hold onto **You**, Your Word, Your promises, and Your character. Thank you for Who You are!

I found notes in my Bible on Ephesians 6 from a Bible study at Restoration Fellowship last year with Pastor Perry Waters. I'll admit when I first heard this perspective, I was taken aback. It was different from what I had been taught. However, the more I reflect on it, the more I realize the truth: We do not put on the armor of God in order to fight. We put it on in order to stand. Jesus already fought all the battles and won! The only place the Word tells me to fight is *"to fight the good fight of faith."* (2Timothy 4:7–8 NIV) The Lord fights my battles! If I fight, then I am not letting the Lord fight. Exodus 14:14 NIV says, *"The Lord will fight for you; you need only to be still."* This was the verse God gave me the night of the stroke, in the ambulance I believe.

I don't fight the devil. He has already been defeated! But my faith is always challenged, and so I must stand in the strength of Jesus inside me and in the authority that He gave me through his name over all forces of evil. (Luke 10:19)

So... resist the devil. See James 4:7 NIV, *"Submit yourselves then to God. Resist the devil and he will flee from you."* First, I must be submitted to God. Only then can I resist the devil. He will flee! Jesus gave us the authority over him.

These reminders about standing have been crucial to me at this time. Perhaps they will be an encouragement to you as well.

October 23, 2014

I will admit that I am weary today. I'm tired of this. Okay? Just being honest. I am not proud of the fact that I get irritated and short with my husband at times. I just want him **back** totally. I'm tired of leading worship without him. I could list a lot of things I'm tired of, but that's just whining so I won't!

So I decided to review the posts from the beginning of this journey. I scrolled all the way down and read them until about August 1. The reminders were **very** obvious of **how far** Brian has come! How much the Lord has done already, how much healing he has received already! We know that this is a process, a long one, quite frankly, **but** God is still in control.

I still believe and am standing on the promise I heard from God those first hours, "This is only a test. He will be totally healed and totally restored." Lately I have heard sermons, come across scriptures, journal entries about standing firm in the Lord. The Holy Spirit knows what we need to hear when we need to hear it. I pray I am always listening.

This reminds me of some of the "lament" psalms from David. He begins at a low point, lists his frustrations, cries out to God…and then ends up in praise and declaration of God's faithfulness and triumph! Amen!

Thank you all for your continued prayers.

*** *Looking back now after three years since this journal entry, I have had many times of the same experience, same types of frustrations. The same method of therapy and mental practice still works: reviewing the faithfulness of God in the past, praising Him for the healing we have received, and trusting Him to continue to be faithful.*

ENCOURAGEMENT

October 25, 2014
Early this morning someone put this inside my car. Yes, Lord! Amen! We receive that encouragement and appreciate it!

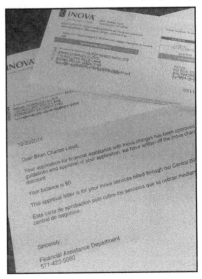

October 27, 2014

7:00 AM ... a brief conversation with a dear friend as she drives to work, giving glory to God for details He is orchestrating, my husband's sense of humor, sunshine highlighting the brilliance of fall colors, and preparing to go for a massage ... all things I am thankful for this Monday morning!

This is the only bill we have seen recently from Brian's week long stay at INOVA ... but the letter came the same day! Praise God! I am sure the actual total bill was well over 100K. God provides!

Just wanted to say what a wonderful time of worship and fellowship, prayer and Word we had together at Fresh Water Fellowship yesterday! I love how the Holy Spirit shows up when we give Him the opportunity to move. He often moves in ways that are unexpected and speaks through people we don't expect. The unity and peace was a true blessing.

Many of you read my posts and knew I had had a rough week. I realized that the bulk of the reason was that I had shifted my focus from Jesus to flesh, from God's long-range perspective onto my frustration with the short-term trial. And while the Lord understands and has grace for our human weariness, the Truth is that we need to encourage ourselves in Him and keep the focus on Christ and stand firm! There were several words of confirmation along these lines yesterday morning at FWF, and I just delighted in seeing the Lord bring it all together.

Pastor Bryan Patrick gave a word before worship relating when he was jumping from airplanes in the military.... How the practice of focusing on a far point on the horizon keeps them from getting motion sickness. Perspective! Brian's OT Friday had used a similar technique. She told him to look **up** while he was walking, not down at the floor. If he picks a point to focus on far in the distance, his center of gravity moves to his chest and gives him more balance and equilibrium. Looking down, our brain doesn't know where we are going and the center of gravity is in our gut. If we start to stumble, we will go right down. Then in one of the worship songs, I had the image of staring at the horizon and one day seeing Jesus revealed coming for us. Now that's perspective!

October 28, 2014

Heading to an attorney this morning to do some pre-eighteen-year birthday stuff regarding Garrett. Also, the neurologist was not satisfied with Brian's custom brace, so we have an appointment this morning for some adjustments. Please pray for both things. Thanks. One of these days I will get to stay home and clean.

Later...

Today was an interesting day. We took Brian's custom brace in to be adjusted since the neurologist wasn't happy with its design. No problem. Will pick it up Thursday.

Then we met with attorneys about things we need to take care of as Garrett comes into adulthood, and also about living wills, power of attorney, and a special needs trust (which is a **crucial** item in regards to special needs children—private message me if you want more info.) We spent two hours at the attorney's office, husband-and-wife tag team who know firsthand the issues since they have one typically developing child and one daughter with Autism. Go figure—the wife used to deal with disability cases, so she gave us a lot of insight and info about that process as well. It was not very encouraging in some ways, **but** it's in God's hands!

After all of that info to process, Brian was a little overwhelmed. (We forget that this is a brain injury, and so at times the stimulation of thoughts, conversations, let alone just the hustle and bustle of being out gets exhausting.) He was feeling rather discouraged. We prayed in the car before going into Wendy's for lunch. He specifically asked for the Lord to give him some encouragement.

Not more than 30 minutes later, a young man walked over to our table and said, "Sir, may I ask why are you walking with a cane?" Brian told him the story as we both took in the fact that he had some obvious issues himself. Then he shared his story with us.... Nearly ten years ago, at twenty-one years old, he was drinking and driving. He was in a terrible accident and suffered multiple injuries, the worst being head trauma. He was in a coma for three years in a wheelchair for two to three years after that, then a walker, a cane, and now walks without any assistance! Part of his skull was removed, and his hands are semi paralyzed due to being in the coma inactive for so long. **And yet** his eyes twinkled and had permanent laugher wrinkle lines as he gave glory to "the good Lord above" for healing him and giving him a second chance. He joined us at the table and we visited for a long while about the Lord, healing processes, and cars. (He's a mechanic too!) He is working part time and driving his own vehicle. A few times he has had the opportunity to share his story at local high schools. Brian said, "Oh, about drinking and driving?" He said, "Well, mainly about perseverance." Wow. I guess so!

Little did he know of Brian's prayer for encouragement. He said he was off work today which was unusual, and he could have eaten at home, but he just had a taste for a Wendy's hamburger. **Yep**! Our God is like that! Do you realize, people, how **much** He loves you? How concerned He is with your every thought?

We got back into our car afterwards feeling refreshed, encouraged, and inspired ... with a new friend and a new shared blessing.

October 29, 2014

This morning ... we have a problem with water drainage at our house which is causing issues with a portion of our basement wall. Today our friend who owns an excavating company is here to fix the problem.

I am eating my breakfast, praying the rain will hold off, and listening to the sound of machinery outside my kitchen window. Asking the Lord what scripture He wants to show me today, I sense Psalm 66 in my spirit ... wow! Awesome!

Psalm 66:1–20 NIV: *Shout for joy to God, all the earth! Sing the glory of his name; make his praise glorious. Say to God, "How awesome are your deeds! So great is your power that your enemies cringe before you. All the earth bows down to you; they sing praise to you, they sing the praises of your name." Come and see what God has done, his awesome deeds for mankind! He turned the sea into dry land, they passed through the waters on foot— come, let us rejoice in him. He rules forever by his power, his eyes watch the nations— let not the rebellious rise up against him. Praise our God, all peoples, let the sound of his praise be heard; he has preserved our lives and kept our feet from slipping. For you, God, tested us; you refined us like silver. You brought us into prison and laid burdens on our backs. You let people ride over our heads; we went through fire and water, but you brought us to a place of abundance. I will come to your temple with burnt offerings and fulfill my vows to you— vows my lips promised and my mouth spoke when I was in trouble. I will sacrifice fat animals to you and an offering of rams; I will offer bulls and goats. Come and hear, all you who fear God; let me tell you what he has done for me. I cried out to him with my mouth; his praise was on my tongue. If I had cherished sin in my heart, the Lord would not have listened; but God has surely listened and has heard my prayer. Praise be to God, who has not rejected my prayer or withheld his love from me!*

October 29, 2014 Brian: "THEN" reflections

Around this time, several months out from the stroke, I was starting to feel better. I wasn't quite so tired all the time. I wanted to get out and do things. Part of the frustration was—and it was a constant reminder—that I knew I couldn't just "go back." Likewise, once you've accepted Christ, once you've sold out to Jesus, you just can't go back. The Spirit won't let you. I'm not saying that prior to the stroke I was involved in any activity that was wrong. It wasn't wrong to be restoring cars or playing guitar. But I just couldn't go back to my way of life, because physically I wasn't able to. David, who owned the shop where I had worked, would call me and ask me to come in and just do little things or consult on a project. I know it was partly just because he was a nice guy as well as my friend, and he was trying to get me back out moving and doing.

Sheila: I think he also wanted you to be able to hold onto your job.

Brian: He was wondering if I was going to come back to work quickly. But part of it is just that he's a decent guy. I would go in once in a while to try to help out, but it was hard. At that point my left hand, arm, and shoulder were really weak, and I was hobbling around on a cane. So I didn't want to be too close to these cars that were worth millions of dollars!

Everybody would invite me out to lunch, which was great. God showed me that I had some really wonderful friends, and great friends in the Lord who loved me. But as much as they wanted to include me and have me come back to who I was—out of the best of intentions on their part—I couldn't. Physically I was unable to, and it wore me out to try.

However, I also knew that I just wasn't supposed to, at that time anyway. I'm not saying that I'll never again do some of the things I did because it wasn't the activity that was wrong. It was partly a heart issue. It was a priorities issue, the way I had put them ahead of God in some ways.

I have to admit, as much as I was all about cars my whole life, the thing that I have missed the most—and it still breaks my heart today—is that I can't play music with my wife. We can't play worship yet like we used to. Now God has been gracious! I'm able to pick up the guitar and play a few little things to soothe my soul, so to speak. And it has progressed, so I can tell that things are still improving. That's one of the ways I can tell I am still gaining and recovering because playing guitar involves very fine motor skills obviously. However I've had to, in some ways, just let that go. I can't think about it too much because it still to this day makes me sad, and I'm two years and nine months out as I write this.

I know that God has told me that someday I will play again, and I will make music for Him, make His music. He'll play through me, so to speak. But it's going to be a different way, a different focus than it was before. I've heard that confirmed from Him several times. It's going to be a way that I didn't see before. I don't know if that means a different way of playing or a different kind of music or what. I don't know what that means yet, but I will someday.

I, like Abraham, just have to believe in God's promises. They are so far out that I can't see them right now. I can't envision them.

I just have to believe what He says. The fact is I know that even if it's not in this lifetime on earth, one day I will sit in a circle with my friends and play guitar again in praise to the Lord. I know that. I can just see us sitting by a tree beside a stream or a river and just playing. Like they did in the blue grass circles—they'd just play whatever they felt led to play. I know I have that promise, that hope.

The point is, we have to be encouraged. Sometimes, the only way that we can be encouraged by God during tough times or in struggles is to look forward—past this life and into the new life with God. Realize that your life is never going to end! Your eternal existence is already set in stone with Jesus. Your spirit will live forever. This temporal body here on this earth may change, and we're going to get a glorified body in our new reality. We will not stop existing! We will be with Christ forever **if** we have chosen to believe in Him. That existence is going to be perfect one day. There's going to be no sin, no pain, no handicaps, no hindrances. We will be perfect with the Lord, and it will be better than anything we can imagine!

*** *As I read this, now three years and three months after the stroke, yes the loss of playing music together is still one of the sharpest to my heart. In fact recently I brought it up to Brian, commenting that he doesn't seem to try to play very much— to "work at it." He said it is not in his heart to do that right now. And he has to trust that when God wants him to do it, He will put the desire in his heart (Psalm 37:4). Otherwise he reiterated that he has had to let it go right now. So difficult for me to hear still! But as he said in the paragraphs above, we both have to hold on to the promises of God and just continue to walk with him.*

CONTINUED RECOVERY

October 30, 2014
Bri doing his stretching exercises this morning. He is asking for prayers. The single most frustration right now is this left shoulder. He lifts it to a certain point and then the pain is so intense that he loses control. Therapists say it is normal pain after a stroke. Please pray for this shoulder as well as his left knee. He feels that if the shoulder and knee would cooperate, everything else would follow. Thank you!

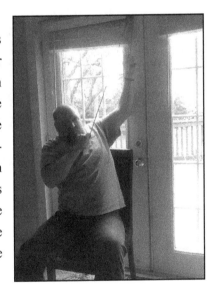

*** *Interesting that just recently (November 2017) he saw our chiropractor out here in Texas about this shoulder issue. The doctor was able to discern what was going on and gave him a great adjustment! We also were blessed to find an excellent deep tissue massage therapist with a background in orthopedics and sports medicine who has been a true catalyst in his continued recovery. There have also been some issues with his right hip and knee due to the massive overcompensation, so he's seeing a physical therapist and incorporating some new exercises. Although*

he often gets frustrated and overwhelmed with the amount of various exercises required on a daily basis, it does seem that the Lord continues to give him improvement and healing, as well as increasing personal discipline.

November 2, 2014

We are moving furniture around today at the Lloyd house ... the daybed is **out** of the living room because Brian has been sleeping upstairs for over a week. Yay! He is negotiating the steps very well.

My mom is coming to stay with us for a while Thursday. We are looking forward to having her here! Please pray that her Social Security comes through. They have been dragging their feet since my dad died (two months ago today.)

November 3, 2014 written by Paula Evans

This morning I was thinking about my friend Brian. He is feeling discouraged regarding his recovery from a stroke. As I was praying for him, his son Garrett popped into my head. Garrett has Down's syndrome and is autistic. And I wondered if this frustration and discouragement Brian feels is a gift, a way to relate to his son that he never had before. His son has always lived with not being the same as everyone else and the frustration of not being able to do what he sees others do with ease. Brian has always been extremely gifted in many ways; there was nothing he couldn't do if he set his mind to it. Now he can't. He is face to face with limitations imposed by his physical body. The opportunity to understand not only his son but others, including me, who are not as quick mentally, or strong physically. We all have value and purpose. We have what we need to do what God has created us for. We have Jesus. The word says in the fourth chapter of Philippians starting at verse 11: *"Not that I speak in respect of want: for I have learned, in whatsoever state I am, therewith to be content. I know both how to be abased, and I know how to abound: everywhere and in all things I am instructed both to be full and to be hungry, both to abound and to suffer need. I can do all things through Christ which strengtheneth me." (KJV)*

BRIAN: Reflections after hearing Paula's entry November 3, 2014, dictated Spring 2017

It reminded me that after I came home and I was kind of hobbling around—I was weak, had the cane, couldn't do things with my left side very much—I could see Garrett watching me. He would watch me with a curious look in his eye as I was trying to do something or pick something up with my left hand but not being able to. He would just be staring at me, almost like, "There's something wrong with Dad. What's wrong?" Then eventually, he would help. He would start putting things over on my right side; or if he saw me struggling to do something with my left side, he would come over and pick it up for me.

I realized that Garrett was making the connection that Dad is hurt on his left side and can't do something, so we need to cater to the strong side. Now, it is a natural approach as a victim to cater everything to your strong side. The danger in that is you start thinking only right-sided to the neglect of your left. You can't do that. You have to force your left side to do things, always a little bit more. Yes, it's very frustrating when you're trying to lift that gallon of milk out of the refrigerator and your hand won't hold it. Your fingers won't hold it, won't pick it up; the wrist won't support it. But you keep trying—helping it with the right hand, making the weak side do a little bit more and a little bit more and a little bit more.

Now, two-and-a-half years later, as I'm observing people around me in daily life, I can spot a stroke victim pretty quickly in public. I can tell by the way they walk—the foot movements or the knee snapping back. Some people have recovered from the stroke effects, and some haven't. Why?

There's the factor of perseverance. I talked to a lady recently who had a stroke twenty-six years ago, and she looked like she had it yesterday. I went over to talk to her because the Lord is highlighting these people to me. (He brings them to my attention, so that I feel drawn to go over to talk to them. I want to see if I'm led to pray for them. I feel like there's a time when God is going to heal people.) When I talked to this lady she was lovely, and her husband was a nice guy as well. Their daughter works locally at the state park, so they come in the restaurant where I help out a few hours per week. They are Christians and love the Lord. The difference is that she gave up on the physical stuff, on trying to get it back. On the other hand, there's a man who works with me who had a stroke six years ago, but you would never know it. He just kept persevering, although he doesn't claim a faith in Jesus.

What's the difference? One person gave up and one didn't. The woman commented on how well I was doing and I just said, "Well, ma'am, it just proves—don't ever give up! Don't ever stop trying because there's still stuff you can get back. God does not mean for us to remain or to be content in staying put. We're to be content no matter where He puts us, but it doesn't mean we're content to stay put."

November 10, 2014

Happy Monday!

Just touching base asking for prayers. I'm recovering from a sinus infection and feel like staying in bed all day ... but no can do. Brian is blessed with another massage this morning, so we are getting ready to go to that.

Bri continues to improve. His shoulder is doing better, and he is able to stretch it out and exercise it more. The new brace is causing some issues with cramming his toe.

I picked up my mom in Breezewood, Pennsylvania, on Thursday, and we are very much enjoying having her here! She is an easygoing, easy-to-please eighty-two-year-old woman, for which I am grateful. We are cozy here in our tight spaces, but we are doing well and enjoying one another.

Some Discouragement
Sets In

November 17, 2014

We are over four months in on this process.

Medicaid has been denied. We are awaiting a final decision on Disability. Brian is gaining a lot of movement but is experiencing quite a bit of pain everywhere on the left side. The doctor and therapists say this is very normal after a stroke. We have been blessed with massages every week from a professional massage therapist who is a friend of ours. Those help him a lot!

Please continue to pray for the Lord's perfect plan in this process, that we would learn everything He wants us to, that we would have **joy**, peace, and patience with one another. The message yesterday was particularly a blessing and encouragement to me... He is our **joy**, Immanuel God with us! Hallelujah!

November 18, 2014

Medicaid denies you if you have over $2,000 of assets.

Now we heard that food stamps will be ending November 30, since Colton's income and my income put us over the limit for a family of four. So frustrating! If we were all just sitting on our butts and not working, we would get help. Something is drastically wrong with the system.

God is in control.

Good news: Brian found his wallet! It's been missing since the night of the stroke. We assumed it had disappeared in transit somewhere. This morning he put a pair of work pants on he hasn't worn in a long time and there it was in the pocket! Lol. I figured it would turn up.

November 20, 2014 PRIVATE JOURNAL

We are four-plus months in on this journey, and I'll admit the wear and tear are showing on me. I have not had normal quiet time or regular exercise. My mom came to stay for two weeks but went home early because she was sick. Although it was nice to have her here, it was added pressure in some ways for me. I've had a couple days when my sugar has crashed, and I have felt awful. Last night was the worst I've experienced for a very long time. We had to miss a leaders' meeting for FWF because I just hit a wall. There was no way I could have gone anywhere.

This is what I wrote about in an email to Aimee: The 24/7 demands are weighing on me, and I seem to be worn down after four-plus months of it. Last night when I was at the lowest, I was just weeping while Brian held me. I said, "I'm tired of being the strong one!" I was immediately convicted that **God** is my strength, and when I am weak **He** is strong. Help me, Jesus. Lord what it is you want to be to me in this time? I feel at this point it has to do with perseverance and long suffering and **joy** in the midst of trial. Contentment.

*** *Looking back, I remember those (frequent) times of just feeling so exhausted—in every way. Physically, emotionally, relationally, spiritually. When I literally felt like I couldn't take another step or make another phone call, or say one more word of encouragement, it was then that Jesus literally bolstered me. The words in 2 Corinthians 12 are "not just idle words for you. They are your life." When I am weak, then I am strong because God's strength is made perfect in my weakness. (2 Corinthians 12:9–10; Deuteronomy 32:47 NIV)*

Now at the time of this writing, three years three months after the stroke, I still experience moments of that kind of exhaustion. In fact, I'm feeling that way right now as I sit on a plane in a waiting pattern on the ground before takeoff. We were scheduled to take off 35 minutes ago. I've been up since 5:30 AM. It's now 7:00 PM and I have a three-plus-hour flight before my head hits the pillow tonight. Just in the last few days I've ridden a roller coaster of emotions from highs of wedding gown shopping with my future daughter-in-law and new therapy improvements for Brian to lows of having to end the life of my beloved furry buddy of ten years. Then, just to pile on, before my first flight today—4 hours ago now—I received word that my mom has to have a breast biopsy tomorrow morning. She's already been through breast cancer twice and is almost eighty-five. The tracks one's mind travels at such news demand fresh commitment to "take every thought captive!" (2 Corinthians 10:5 NIV)

What's the answer? What is the hope? What source can I tap into for strength and peace as well as stamina for the rest of today, not to mention what may or may not lie ahead? The answer is the same today as it was November 2014. Jesus. My Rock. My Hope. My Strength. As that old hymn says, "I don't know what tomorrow holds, but I know Who holds tomorrow." Mom said earlier, "My friend—who is rather a worrywart—admired my faith and calmness facing this development. I told her, 'Well, we either believe God or we don't. He's not going to leave me now.'" Amen.

November 24, 2014

Haven't posted in a while. I must admit that I have struggled with discouragement the last few weeks. Have also not been in top health, which doesn't help. However, I had a 'Come to Jesus' meeting this morning during my quiet time. (That's another thing—I hadn't been as diligent about going out to the studio and having my quiet time each day. I would read couple verses but just not spending the quality time with the Lord in study, prayer, and worship.) It's easy to find excuses not to, **but** it greatly affects our attitude and perspective.

The last two Sundays we have heard particularly good words of encouragement through sermons. November 16 at FWF was about

THE JOY OF THE LORD IS MY STRENGTH (Nehemiah 8:10 NIV)…so to walk around in discouragement and despair is actually a sin of unbelief saying that we don't believe God is who He says He is and that He can do what He says He can do. Forgive me, Lord!

Now, yes, I believe that the Lord understands that we are but dust, and He is gracious and compassionate when we are going through trials. However, He gave us His word as encouragement, and He also laid it on our hearts at the beginning of this journey that Brian would be fully restored and healed through faith in Jesus' name. Brian knew from the start that the Lord has things to teach him through the process. Well, the process is ongoing. Duh. That's why it's called a process. So, Lord, thank you for your graciousness, but I pray that You would give me **Your** strength and **Your** joy to continue to walk through this journey and not give in to the enemy's darts of discouragement.

Yesterday's sermon was about being **thankful** and counting our blessings! Truly we have **so much** to be thankful for! Lord, deliver me from all discouragement and fill those vacated places with your Spirit and with an attitude of gratitude and joy. **Thank You!**

Just thought I would be honest… perhaps someone else needs to hear it too.

November 24, 2014

BRIAN: THEN… reflections on Nebuchadnezzar, Job… how long the trials lasted, and the root of Who God is.

At this point we're four-and-a-half months after the stroke. That's enough time that you start thinking, "Okay, God, this has been long enough." We started to get frustrated. "Why can't I get over this? Why can't God just heal me?" In response, I went back to a story my friend John and I read while I was in the residential rehab center in Winchester, Virginia.

John would come up to see me every Sunday morning, and we'd have worship right there out on the courtyard. One of the things we read was the story of Nebuchadnezzar from Daniel 4.

Nebuchadnezzar, the great king of Babylon, walks out onto his balcony overlooking the city and boasts, "Look at this great city that I have made with my own hands!" God prophesied to him through Daniel some time earlier, telling the king that unless he changed his ways and acknowledged that "Heaven rules," he would be struck down and would live like the wild animals for seven years.

Nebuchadnezzar did not change his ways and immediately upon making that boastful statement he became like a wild beast, lost his sanity, was removed from his kingdom, and lived out with the cattle for seven years. He ate grass! The Bible says that his hair became like feathers and his fingernails like the claws of a bird. And he lived like that for seven years. Seven years! We were four months in and getting frustrated. Seven years he did that. And then finally he acknowledged the Lord and everything was restored.

I look at Job, all the hardships he went through, how long it lasted, and what he endured. Then he acknowledged God—he always had acknowledged God, but through his trials he truly came to the root of Who God is—His awesomeness, His mighty power, His majesty. Job came face to face with the completeness of God, the overwhelming power in what God controls and what He does. (See Job chapters 38–42) In admitting that, and in praying for his friends, Job was restored to a greater status than he had been before. But it took years. It wasn't just four months. We have to endure something for two weeks and we get frustrated.

God was showing me these truths at that point in our journey. God was speaking to my heart, "Yes this is going to be a longer process than you would like, but you will be restored once you come to the point I need you to come to."

I can tell you right now (April 2017) that I'm not done. The more He shows me, the more I realize the issues of flesh versus the Spirit. Gratifying the flesh has been ingrained in me since I was born. The world tells you, "You need to be this way, do this, have this, buy this, strive for this...." The "all about me philosophy" is ingrained in us from the time we're little kids. (Isaiah 47:10 NIV sums it up perfectly with the motto from the Babylonian empire, which throughout Scripture is a model of rebellion against the Lord. *"I am, and there is none besides me!"*)

Sheila: Yes, because it's a fallen world.

Brian: I'm not saying it was my parents' fault or that they did anything wrong. It's just the indoctrination of our culture: what you see on TV, billboards, media, advertising, magazines, what you learn in school, what your friends teach you about. We hear the popular old sayings, "You have to pull yourself up by your bootstraps. There's no such thing as a free lunch." Some of that is true while we live here in this world.

But the fact is God wants to be involved in every area of our life. He wants to lead us in every aspect of our life. We must rely on Him totally, let Him tell us what we need to know. I am a slave to Christ. As I am made a slave to Christ, I give up my rights—to everything. I have no rights on my own. I have no "self-determination" anymore. Oddly enough, when we learn that, we experience true freedom! That's where the freedom lies. Because now it's not up to me. It's not relying on me. It's not thinking, "If something doesn't work, it's because I failed." No, I trust in God for everything. And He shows me what He allows me or wants me to do.

That's a hard one. I'm still learning that, still battling that, and I don't know if I'll ever be truly done with that until I see Him face to face. But I do know that's what He wants me to learn more fully—that I have no rights. He never promises us happiness. He never promises us prosperity in the world. We are prosperous in Him. We have the joy of Him. We have the promise of Him and the abundance of the Spirit because that's what matters. This worldly stuff—what does the Word say? It passes away. Moth and rust destroy. (Matthew 6:19–20) It doesn't last; it's temporary. That's all the devil can offer you—stuff that won't last. That's why you always want more because it doesn't last; it doesn't truly satisfy. So we think, if I get more—of whatever—then I'll have enough to see me through. And that's a lie. Jesus is enough to see us through! He doesn't deteriorate. His promises don't whither. What He gives us lasts. As He told the Samaritan woman at the well, *"Those who drink the water I give will never be thirsty again."* (John 4:13–14 TLB) Conversely, what the enemy offers makes you more thirsty, makes you crave more.

When you drink of Christ you can be fully satisfied. For eternity.

Decision to praise 11/25/14. Oftentimes we have to make a conscious decision to **do so!**

Thanksgiving night was the first time Brian was able to make some sounds on the guitar! Thank you, Lord! I finished a new stained glass piece that God gave me the idea for. It is indicative of new thing, new beginning, and a Southwest feel!

November 25, 2014

Brian's OT today figured out the problem with his shoulder! She isolated it and gave him some simple exercises to do! **Yeah!** Thank you, Lord, for encouragement! Also, he is feeling confident to drive short distances which I know has got to feel wonderful!

One of the things I so appreciate about the Psalms is that through them, David pours out his heart to the Lord. We read the full range of emotions: ecstatic praise, deep despair, laments and frustrations, desire for judgement on his enemies, discouragement, proclamations of peace and security, and more.

Today I was led to flip through the Psalms and make notes of the verses where he says I **will praise, I will sing**. There are many! But here are a few: Psalm 9:1–2; 27:6b; 34:1–8; 50:23; 57:7–9; 59:16–17; 63:2–5,7; 71:14; 119:171–172; 146:1–2 (all NIV)

I was doing some yard work outside and literally this happened … *"He put a new song in my mouth, a hymn of praise to our God."* (Psalm 40:3 NIV). Into the studio I went and sat down at the piano.

BRIAN'S TESTIMONY VIDEO recorded on November 27, 2014

Hello and Happy Thanksgiving!

Sheila wanted me to do this again. She wants to put another video of me on Facebook.

But anyway....

It's Thanksgiving Day, a time for everybody to reflect and remember our blessings. I'm going to say it's time to reflect on what God has given us, because it's all His anyway. I'm thankful for what God lets me have. He let me have more time here. I could have gone home to be with Him and been happy, but I'm here and I'm happy because I'm happy with whatever God gives me. Ultimately it's all about Him and not about me. We want to make it about us. We want to believe the lie that somehow we deserve it or that we're entitled to something. And that's not true. We're entitled to whatever He gives us. To some He gives a lot and to some He gives a little. It's all about Him and His Son, Jesus Christ. That's what I'm thankful for—my Savior! He gave His life for us so that we could have eternal life and not be a slave to sin anymore.

So that's what I'm thankful for this Thanksgiving Day! [He waves goodbye to the camera with his left hand that has the I AM SECOND bracelet on it.]

November 28, 2014

Another interesting day in the Lloyd household. Brian has been having very severe headaches behind his right eye for four days on and off. Trip to ER. Been here 3 1/2 hours. IV dilaudid hardly touched the pain. CT scan showed sinusitis! They are treating that with strong antibiotics and recommending follow up with ENT next week. We are just grateful that it is not stroke related, for good care and for an answer! Would have been more fun to do Christmas decorating.

Answers ... and The Beginning
of A New Process

December 1, 2014

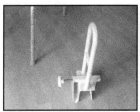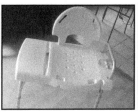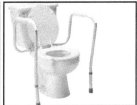

Praise God, Brian is **done** with these things! Does anyone need them? I would like them **gone** ASAP.

First one is a handle that will fit on a regular tub side. Second is obviously a chair for the shower. Third are lightweight handles for over any toilet.

December 2, 2014
Brian has been looking at Joshua, Gideon, etc. in the Bible. They were totally convinced what God had said. What are we convinced about?

December 2, 2014 Evening
Left home at 8:15 AM this morning. Got home at 3:00 PM. Doctor appointments, exam, shot for sinus infection for Bri... potential sinus

surgery of some sort. Unrelated to stroke stuff as far as we know. Now teaching for five hours. Whew! I'm tired! **But** thankful for answers and trusting the Lord is making him better than new—figuring out what's been causing these terrible headaches this past week. Please continue to pray for our strength, financial provision, and our ability to put ourselves in a position to hear the Lord. Thank you.

We have to turn around and go back up to Winchester tomorrow for a recheck after the shot of antibiotics. Then at 1:40 PM he sees an orthopedist in Woodstock to rule out rotator cuff injury. It's a week of appointments!

FB post December 2

Well, I am tired tonight **but** have to share a praise report. We are continually blown away by the favor and blessing of God!

Heard this afternoon that the 100 percent financial aid letter we received from INOVA might not be valid. Sat on hold 40 minutes. Finally talked to a very kind financial manger at INOVA. We had actually qualified for only 80 percent but someone made a mistake and sent us the wrong letter! So....they have to honor it! She told me that any bills we receive, we just send them a copy of the letter. Not more than 2 hours later Brian got a call from a bill collector. He explained and the man said, "Oh yes, I am just seeing that in the system. Sorry, Mr. Lloyd!"

I had explained to the woman about our current financial situation, but then I had added, "God is taking care of us. He is so good." She said, "He is indeed!"

Amazing. Thank you, Father! We sit today facing the real possibility that Brian might have to have sinus surgery (consultation at UVA, University of Virginia Medical Center, next week), and although that is a little overwhelming... the thought of more medical bills, more time I will need to take off work... this reminder of provision and grace comes tonight. And He will continue providing because that is Who He is.

December 4, 2014

Another interesting day yesterday ... recheck with ENT. Brian was feeling **much** better, looked better, and said he felt overall "brighter." No headache all day! This was the first pain-free day since November 24. Praise God! The ENT says UVA sinus professor is the one who will consult with us next week and decide procedure, but it is important to have that done because the distorted sinuses are pressing up against his right eye. No wonder he's been having so much pain!

We want to highly recommend this ENT if you need one ... Doctor Peter Johnson in Winchester, VA. Not only is he a very good doctor but he is a strong believer in Jesus Christ. We had a wonderful conversation together ... the doctor was basically preaching a little sermon. He began with, "I am a student of the Bible...." We said, "So are we," and we were off. What a blessing and encouragement that was!

Yesterday afternoon Brian also saw an orthopedist for his shoulder. Although part of the exam showed symptoms typical for stroke pain, there were also aspects indicative of rotator cuff injury. Upon reflection, Brian said that shoulder has bothered him for years. The doctor ordered an MRI next week and we'll go from there.

The Lord is getting him all fixed up! The next stage of our lives in ministry is going to be fun ... and quite different, we have a feeling. Please pray that we hear the Lord clearly and follow Him well.

December 5, 2014

Saw a cardiologist yesterday for a consultation/follow up. They did EKG right there in the office and then read those in comparison with EKG and Echograms done at INOVA right after the stroke. The doctor said Brian's heart looks strong and besides maintaining the meds, good diet, exercise, he doesn't think we need to do anything further about heart stuff!

At the same time as the stroke, they said he had a "mild heart attack," and yet there was **no** damage done to the heart. The doctor gave us a very detailed explanation, but the conclusion was that what Brian suffered was **not** a heart attack induced by a blood clot. The enzymes that had been detected, which the EMT guys detected, were just released by the heart due to the stress from the stroke. But he did **not** have a heart attack. A heart attack can release those enzymes, but in his case it was just that the heart was pumping fast from the stress of the stroke.

Good news! Once again, thank you, Lord!

Just in the last week he has seen/been to … ER, ENT twice, hospital for antibiotic injection, physical therapy, fitted for a new knee brace, orthopedist to examine his shoulder, and the cardiologist … good grief! **But** thankful that we are getting all these issues resolved.

December 6, 2014

Today we actually just did something **fun** … visited a couple flea markets. Spent $13 bucks on a couple cool things and just enjoyed being together. It felt like a vacation!

December 11, 2014

What is your identity? The world offers answers in many forms: you are your looks, your status, your income, your talent. The Bible offers deeper, lasting, and more satisfying answers. If we know Jesus Christ, then we are *"a chosen people, a royal priesthood, a holy nation, a people belonging to God!"* (1 Peter 2:9–10 NIV). Do a word study in the New Testament on the phrase "in Christ" and see for yourself the amazing qualities which describe our identity! Lord, help us live according to our identity, not our circumstances.

*** *Accepting, believing, and walking in my identity in Christ has been a major growing edge for me the last several years. The details of that are a much longer discussion, probably even another book topic! However, it is summed up well in a poem the Lord gave me a few months ago. See Appendix.*

MRI on shoulder Tuesday. We'll get results tomorrow.

Today going to UVA for consult with a sinus professor … looks like a beautiful day for a drive. Thankful we enjoy being together! After five weeks apart when he was in the hospital, God has redeemed the time.

Yesterday marked five months on this journey! Wow. Can't believe it. Certainly was **not** what we had planned for this time, but God had other ideas. He works **all** things for good!

Isaiah 55:8–11 NIV: *"For my thoughts are not your thoughts, neither are your ways my ways," declares the Lord. "As the heavens are higher than the earth, so are my ways higher than your ways and my thoughts than your thoughts. As the rain and the snow come down from heaven, and do not return to it without watering the earth and making it bud and flourish, so that it yields seed for the sower and bread for the eater, so is my word that goes out from my mouth: It will not return to me empty, but will accomplish what I desire and achieve the purpose for which I sent it."*

From Aimee Patrick: Most of you have been keeping updated on the Facebook page with Brian and Sheila. His progress is amazing... God gets all the Glory and all the Praise from both Brian and Sheila.

They are going into the fifth month of the Season that God has so graciously given them! With that being said, I wanted to post some family and financial updates. Their SNAP (food stamp) benefits ended in November. These benefits were taking care of most of their groceries. Medicaid has been denied, which would have covered balances on medical bills. Some of the bills have been covered by insurance and others under financial aid. However, there are a few that have balances after both of these items have been reviewed.

Social Security Disability rating is still pending. And the household bills are still coming in. Sheila has been attempting to keep her piano schedule as full as she can, along with taking Brian and Garrett to different doctor appointments, therapy, consultations, etc. They have been traveling anywhere from Edinburg, Woodstock, to Winchester, and then today as far as UVA for the latest concern with Brian's sinuses.

I reopened this YOUCARING.com site for a few reasons. ONE - For continued **prayer** for Brian, Sheila, Colton, and Garrett and all the medical professionals whom they will see. TWO - To remind us that we are all blessed. THREE - To bring everyone up to date and see where you can help. It's an ongoing process for them from the healing of the stroke, to a lifestyle change, seasonal change, as well as a financial change for them.

Brian is building models as therapy for his left hand. Zeppelin is checking just in case it's actually food!

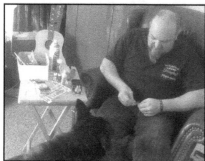 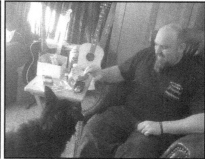

Helicopter ride from Winchester ER to INOVA, Fairfax, the night of the stroke was $41,000. Anthem has been dragging their feet paying and finally denied the claim, saying that Brian didn't get preauthorization! Really?! Yes, we didn't plan ahead very well. Lol. The rep from the air care company says they are actually breaking federal law now, so she is filing formal complaints. Please pray for justice as the Lord wants it to work out.

This bill, along with about $1,500 owed on others are the **only** bills left unpaid from the whole five-week ordeal. Praise God! Subsequent therapy still going on are covered by the financial aid we have received from Valley Health and INOVA. Oh! I wrote one check for $6.11 to a radiology company for something.

Now, it looks like we'll start again with UVA for the sinus stuff... and rotator cuff surgery **if** that is necessary. God is making him better than new to prepare him for the next phase the Lord has for us in ministry. Go, God!

December 11, 2014 lots of time to write as we're sitting in waiting rooms for hours.

Another long day but more answers and more signs of the Lord's blessing.

We left home at noon and returned around 8:45 PM. Consult with professor of sinus surgery at UVA. We saw Brian's CT scans from the night of the stroke as well as November 28. I'll spare you the graphic (and gross) details of mucus seals, etc.... suffice it to say that **yes**, it appears he has had messed up sinuses for probably years. It is imperative that they are repaired. And so surgery is scheduled for January 28, 2015 at UVA. It is **not** the nightmare sinus surgery we've heard about with the miles of packing up your nose etc., etc. Certainly it won't be a picnic, but it should allow him to feel **lots** better!

*** *I remember that day clearly! We met with the top sinus professor/ surgeon at the University of Virginia Medical Center, Doctor Payne. On the drive over, Brian said to me, "Honey, I really do not want to undergo sinus surgery! I've gone through so much already." Of course I could agree! I said, "Let's just pray and trust that God will make it really clear what needs to be done." Sitting in the doctor's exam room later, he popped Brian's CT scan up on the computer. It looked like a negative of a skull as you might expect, with one major alteration—it appeared as though there was a big third eyeball in between his two eye sockets! The doc explained that this was a mucus plug that was pushing against his right eye socket. It was actually changing the shape of his right eye. Left uncorrected it would continue to grow and eventually push the eye out of its socket altogether! Gee. Pretty clear answer! Brian said, "That would be inconvenient at parties. Please pass the —uh ... oh. Please pass me my eyeball!" His sense of humor has been a saving grace more times than I can count.*

After the doctor's office, we checked in at the hospital and met with the anesthesiology RN so we'll be all set.

We arrived home, checked the mail, and found

1) denial from Social Services for heating assistance;
2) anniversary card with an Olive Garden gift card; and
3) groceries dropped off by a friend and a beautiful card with some cash in it too! **Thank You, Lord!**

A VERY DIFFERENT
HOLIDAY SEASON

This Christmas season is unlike any we have experienced before. Our twenty-fourth wedding anniversary is Monday December 15. I am one of these sappy, twinkly-light-loving, music enthusiast, tradition-embracing, goody-cooking, pretty-presents wrapper, and elaborate decorator, Elouise book and all! This year, although I still see the beauty in it all, we are definitely taking a much simpler, low-key approach... enjoying the season but mainly just appreciating one another and the true meaning— EMMANUEL (God with us!)

December 13, 2014

Doesn't need rotator cuff surgery, thank God. MRI doesn't seem to be a tear, just bone spurs. Probably because of weakness on left side due to stroke is why he's feeling it more. There is some cartilage stress and inflammation, but doctor felt with everything else going on we didn't need to do anything about it right now. We'll check back in a few months. **Grateful** we don't have to add that to the list right now!

A blessing today...

The Medical Transport Service (ambulance which drove Brian from INOVA to Winchester Rehab 7/18) was charging about $640. They said Valley Health financial aid didn't cover it and we were responsible—interest-free, whatever monthly payments we could make until it was paid off. I sent in a check for $20 last week.

Today I received that check back from them along with a letter saying, "After discussions about our current situation, we qualify for the 'hardship' category." They are waiving the entire fee. Thank you, Lord!

December 18, 2014

We enjoy receiving Christmas cards from friends far and wide this time of year. Many of them have photos and/or letters summing up highlights of the past year. I must admit that it is with mixed emotions that I read them this year. Our past five-and-a-half months have been **so very** different!

This excerpt from a dear friend's (I couldn't remember who to ask permission to share it) letter touched my heart: *"I quickly realized that this indeed would be a different Christmas and being the 'traditionalist' that I am, it came with bittersweet tears and emotions. However, through the a song on the radio called "A Different Christmas", God quickly reminded me that although it may be a different Christmas, it is Christmas just the same! God came, God lives, and God forever will remain. This is the message of Christmas. Whether we celebrate in our living rooms, hospital rooms, nursing homes, God will meet us wherever we are. Sometimes taking that road to Bethlehem in our hearts isn't always easy. It is our wish and prayer that wherever you celebrate Jesus' birth it will be glorious!"*

Amen. Let it be.

December 21, 2014

Just wanted to share some praises:

Our church family blessed us with an anniversary gift, so we celebrated last night with dinner and a live show: *A New Christmas Carol*. What a nice evening! A surprise little hole in the wall place that showcased some very nice talent, of all ages. That's one of our favorite stories ... as Brian says, "A true story of redemption."

In the last couple days we've received Christmas cards with

unexpected blessings inside... Food Lion gift card, Olive Garden gift card, Sheetz gift card, and cash. God is so good! We are planning to head to PA for a few days after Christmas and the expenses always add up. Thank you, Father, for your provision, and thanks to those through whom He gives.

Merry Christmas! God is with **all** of us! Emmanuel

Recorded December 25, 2014

He's been saying he wanted a shirt like this since August so...

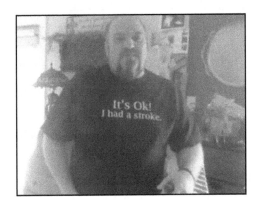

Merry Christmas everybody! Just saying something for the holidays. Got my new shirt for Christmas— hoping it still applies. It gets me a lot of free meals, really good service, seats right by the door at restaurants.

Sheila: Because you don't have the four-prong cane anymore.

Brian: Well, I had the four-prong cane but I don't need it anymore. The walking stick doesn't really help much. People think that's just decoration. Know that whatever you're going through, whether it seems good or bad, God is good. God is there. He is on the throne. He has not forsaken you. He will never leave you. If He puts something in front of you, He gives you a way through it. God doesn't always deliver us from the problem, but He delivers us through the problem. The Israelites had to go through the Red Sea. They didn't get transported to the other side magically. But God provided a way for them to make it through. He will provide a way for you to make it through. And we all have Jesus on the other side waiting for us. Remember God is still good and you can find joy in the midst of whatever you are going through. Thanks.

January 1, 2015 New Year's Day reflections in PRIVATE JOURNAL
While Brian was still in rehab, my ninety-eight-and-a-half-year-old father declined in health and died August 2, 2014. The mixture of emotions in me through this time is difficult to put into words. I was so thankful that Brian and I had made the trip to New Castle, PA, on Memorial Day 2014 and July 4, because obviously he did not get to come to the funeral. Colton drove me and my mother-in-law, Wanda Lloyd, up for the funeral in August. It was a very refreshing time for me actually. I am so blessed with such a wonderful godly, loving family! And it was balm for my soul to be with them at that time. To celebrate a life well lived and well loved.

Christmas night we traveled up to New Castle, PA, to spend some time with my mom and extended family. Part of the celebration was for my niece Dawn Mooney's bridal shower (wedding in May with Joe Mondry, whom we are thrilled to welcome into the family!).

A big part of my desire for the weekend was to help my mom sort through my dad's files and desk. For anyone who knew dad's "den," you know what a **huge** job that is! We did really get **a lot** done...trips to Salvation Army and several to the dumpster! I think that dear man never threw anything away! As a friend reminded me, he was a man of his time—living through the Depression and several wars, one learned to **save** things "just in case" and also to document **thoroughly**. Well, then, my dad was a pro. lol.

Here are a couple of my favorite finds which made me just scratch my head: a brown lunch bag with my brother Kevin's name in sharpie marker written on it. Inside was a broken metal top of an electric razor. Next to it was another piece (battery?) of that razor with a Post-it note taped to it. The Post-it note was taped down and dated twice along with the words, "Replaced the blades in Kevin's razor."

His old leather wallet. In the clear window insert was a piece of a notecard with the date along with "Saturday... transferred the contents into new wallet."

About a dozen spines (**just** the spines) of checkbooks rubber banded together.

But along with these strange items were countless others that warmed my heart... hundreds of cards given to him by family and friends for various occasions, pictures of my boys when they were little, scraps of notebook paper where he jotted down scripture verses he was studying or notes from sermons. (One in particular said, "Romans 5—see first 5 verses." Yep! I agree, Dad, pretty awesome.) Over everything his distinctive, beautiful handwriting dating items or noting who things were from, etc.

I also found a wonderful article from a couple decades ago about the Mooney Family Reunion, the year we included a fiftieth anniversary celebration for Uncle Bill and Aunt Rose. In it, details were shared of my grandfather's immigration to America from Italy around the turn of the twentieth century and some wise advice to his six sons. Made me realize once again how a family can give us grounding and a sense of identity. **And yet** how much greater is the grounding and identity, sense of belonging that we can **all** have in Jesus despite our family of origin.

I knew that this job of cleaning out was one I wanted to do. It is a part of the grieving for me, tender memories. Heart full of gratitude for the man God gave me as a father. Not perfect, but one who left quite a heritage.

January 3, 2015

Happy New Year everyone! Garrett and I have been struggling with the sinus/cold/flu yuck **but** thankfully Brian and Colton have been healthy. Please pray that Brian stays healthy in preparation for the sinus surgery January 28. Thanks.

January 8, 2015

"In this world you will have trouble, but take heart, I have over-come the world!"...Jesus, king of Kings, **author** of **life**. John 16:33 NIV

UVA has denied our application for financial assistance for Brian's sinus surgery January 28. I'm very surprised, and we are going to try to appeal. But I guess we will get to see the Lord work a different way!

I am reminding myself today that I am not waiting on disability decision/income or even Brian's physical restoration. I am waiting on the **Lord**. His character and timing are completely trustworthy. He is faithful!

Sixth-Month Mark

January 10, 2015

Today is the sixth-month mark. Wow.

This has been the most difficult thing we have faced in our lives. The only thing to which I can compare it is when Garrett was diagnosed with Down's syndrome at one week old. My world was rocked, and I embarked on a journey of intense growth (and healing from wounds I didn't realize I had due to growing up with a brother who has Down's.) However, adjusting to parenting a special needs child was something we stood together solidly as partners. Brian was truly the strong one during that time!

During this season, though, we are still standing together as partners. It's just different. Am I ready for this process to be over? **Yes!** Do I want my husband "back"— totally strong and restored? **Yes!** And **yet**, I have to say honestly that the Lord has taught us **so much** during these six months. *"Because of the Lord's great love we are not consumed. His mercies are new every morning. Great is Your faithfulness!"* (Lamentations 3:25 NIV)

God has strengthened our marriage, deepened our love and appreciation for one another, and most importantly shown us more about who **He** is as our Provider, Sustainer, Strength, and Shield.

All of us in life face challenges and difficulties. But it is during these times that we are refined. Often it is during the tough times when we experience the most growth and maturity by the grace of God and by our willingness to surrender to His plan. I am not saying that God causes bad things to happen. We live in a fallen world. Bad things do happen. However, the Lord promises to work *"All things together for **good** for those who love him and are called according to His purpose."* (Romans 8:28 NIV, emphasis mine) **Only** God can turn what Satan meant for our harm and turn it into a blessing.

January 12, 2015

I posted Saturday that it was the six-month mark since the stroke. Although I shared some of the emotional and spiritual insights, I did not share how he is doing physically! So... Brian is able to walk all around without any cane, even outside! The left hand has **much** more movement and strength. His shoulder doesn't hurt like it did, and he is able to work out with it. His walking is more smooth and the left knee doesn't "snap" as badly as it did before. He is cleared to drive! This past week he traveled to Ohio with a missionary friend of ours, and he drove for hours at a time even through Columbus. Brian commented that he had to concentrate more on driving than he used to, but he felt comfortable and competent. He noticed afterwards that he was mentally tired... after all, his brain is still healing. We forget that this was actually a brain injury, therefore healing takes time.

Current **prayer** requests physically... pray that his left ankle and foot would have full range of motion. Also, pray that his left hand/fingers would continue to gain dexterity and strength. Pray that he would be able to play the guitar back to—and exceeding—what he used to. He **is** able to play a little bit, but needs the speed and dexterity to change chords more quickly. Also, please pray for his sinus surgery at UVA January 28 (which is not stroke-related) but in desperate need. And continue to pray for however the Lord wants to meet our financial needs. We are still waiting to hear from Disability.

Thank You!

January 13, 2015

Thanks to our friend Michael Link who not only makes my husband laugh hysterically, but who is also an avid weight/athletic trainer. He is here helping Brian develop a workout plan. One recommendation is getting him a roller fitness ball ... I will post a pic ... wondering if anyone has one they do not need before we buy one from eBay.

January 16, 2015

Another example of the Lord's provision occurred today ... and I just want to say that I don't share these things to sound super spiritual. We share them because God is showing Himself to be **real** to us over and over again on this journey, and we believe part of the reason for that is so that we can bear witness.

Anyway ... today our dear friend Aimee Patrick shared at her home school meeting in Winchester about the Pampered Chef fundraiser. She was thinking maybe a few of the ladies would want to buy raffle tickets for one of the special items. Well, woman after woman came up to her saying they didn't really need any PC but they just wanted to give us money. What is the total? $635! From a group of people who don't know us from Adam.

Then Aimee said, "How much was your SNAP benefits (food stamps) per month?" I answered, "$632."

Notice that the Lord supplied more than the "world" would have supplied. There's a lesson in that. Kingdom math is different.

Once again we just say, "Thank you, Lord."

Also today I totally screwed up our appointment time for Brian's OT therapy in Woodstock. We just were hanging out at the house all day, relaxing and taking it easy. I was positive that our appointment was at 2:30—so positive in fact that I never even double-checked my calendar. We walk in 7 minutes early ... only to find out that our appointment had been 1:45 PM! His OT, Amy Gray, said she had been concerned about us because we had never no-showed. She was kind enough to see us after her last client at 3:15 PM. It's more like visiting with a friend by now anyway! The three of us chat about all kinds of stuff while she presents Brian with new challenges for his fine motor development in each session.

January 18, 2015
We were blessed with a couple big boxes of groceries yesterday! The items we weren't able to use or didn't need we were able to pass along to a friend who was in need. It's cool when God multiplies!

January 20, 2015
Finally have the house all to myself for a few hours!

Had some good time of personal worship out in the studio. Then was led to just curl up on the couch and imagine the arms of my Abba Father surrounding me.

Three scriptures, in particular, came to mind: how the Holy Spirit intercedes for me with groans that words can't express (Romans 8:26–27 NIV); the Lord singing over me (Zephaniah 3:17 NIV); and the Lord surrounding me with songs of deliverance (Psalm 32:7 NIV). Amen.

*** *Looking back, what I did that day I often do in a variety of ways—a walk in the woods or at the park, driving without any music playing in the car, sitting in my favorite chair at home and enjoying total silence. There is such a lesson in taking time alone to bask in the Lord's presence! I'm convinced that there are so many times that He wants to speak to us, but we are not still or quiet enough to listen. Some people are afraid of being alone and find silence uncomfortable. But God often speaks not in the whirlwind or the thunder, but in the still small Voice. I would encourage you to be willing to wait in silence until you hear Him.*

January 24, 2015
THANK you to all of those who placed a Pampered Chef order during the fundraiser for us! Total sales were just over $1,100!

January 24, 2015

Sooooo glad to have Brian back up with us! Bass takes a little less finger movement….

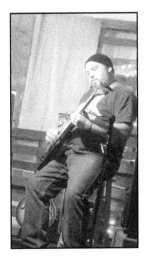

January 25, 2015

Brian has been building models to help with his hand. He's wanting some more. Anyone know of some sources that are fairly inexpensive? We've gotten them so far at Hobby Lobby. Obviously he likes the vintage ones.

FIRST SINUS SURGERY

January 28, 2015

I am sitting in the UVA cafeteria while Brian is having his sinus surgery, and I'm reading the chronological bible for January 28. It is Exodus 23 where the Lord is setting up the groundwork of His covenant with the Israelites. As He was describing the nations they would conquer, He said, *"I will not drive them out in a single year."* God goes on to explain the reasons behind this ... the land would become desolate and wild animals would overtake. He says, *"Little by little I will drive them out before you until you have increased enough to take possession of the land." (Exodus 23:29–30 NIV)*

It was a reminder to me to trust the Lord in this process.

How many times have we wanted this to be over? How many times have we thought, "Okay, can we be done with this journey and on to the new thing?" Plenty. But God made it clear to Brian at the beginning that this would be a process, and Brian willingly surrendered to the process because he knew that in it were lessons and growth. A long time ago we both surrendered and made Jesus the Lord of our lives (not just our Savior) ... consequently, He's in charge.

In the Israelites' best interest, the Lord did not drive out all their enemies in one fell swoop although, certainly, He was capable of doing so. Okay. Lord. We trust you.

January 29, 2015

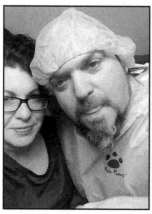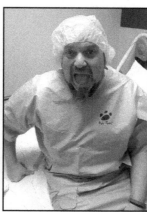

Wow! I feel like I have my husband back! It's amazing the change! Even as soon as last night. The sinus surgery was over around 1:30 PM. Took him a while to wake up from anesthesia. I went up at 4:15 PM and we left UVA around 5:15 PM.

Also, he said he notices that he is not craving sugar and junk. We remember way back in ICU at Fairfax when the doctor came in and suggested sleep apnea for the first time. He said what happens is your body isn't getting oxygen, so you crave carbs, you gain weight, the heart is under stress and—Bam!—stroke. Brian (through very slurred speech) at the time said, "That sounds like my life." Well, thank you Lord that we have found the problem!

As of 6:30 AM he is up and feeling great, going to meet a friend for breakfast. He is driving because he's had **no** pain and **no** pain meds! Not even Tylenol.

Here's a word from Brian this morning! He can feel his body being rejuvenated! Thank you, Lord!

January 29, 2015 Recorded morning after first sinus surgery:

Brian: I had my surgery yesterday. Other than a sore throat from the breathing tube with the anesthesia, I'm feeling amazing! I feel badass and booger-free! This is just another example that God is good. God takes what the enemy meant for evil and uses it for good. (Genesis 50:30 and Romans 8:28)

Because of the stroke, they discovered this huge sinus problem. I'm being made better than I ever was, so thank you Lord! I can rejoice even in the midst of suffering, so thank you Lord. That's really all I have to say. I can breathe—through my nose!

Sheila: Oxygen is a good thing!

Brian: Oxygen is not overrated!

I, on the other hand, am going back to bed and am looking forward to a quiet morning! It's been a very long couple days. But the boost to my spirit in seeing him this improved is the main thing I needed. I was feeling pretty down last night. I got him home at 7:20 PM and then went out to Walmart to get his meds. Got home at 8:30 PM and took care of Colton who had the stomach bug all day. Went to bed just feeling so "at the end" in every way. What an encouragement to hear Brian this morning and see his personality back! Oh, thank you, Father.

BRIAN
January 29, 2015 LOOKING BACK
The first sinus surgery was a major thing! The day after, actually even coming home from surgery, even though I was sore and kind of out of it, I wasn't in pain like I expected. I immediately felt better because the headache was finally gone! (I had had a terrible headache since about Thanksgiving.) And, boy, I slept that night! I woke up at 6:30 AM feeling even better than when I'd first put the CPAP machine on during my sleep study. I hadn't slept that well in years! I was awake. I didn't have to have coffee and sugar to wake me up. I was ready to go. Now, I did have some coffee at breakfast just because I like coffee!

While I was driving to meet a friend for breakfast, I noticed I was more alert, brighter, driving easier, steadier…it was just miraculous! The surgeon from UVA was amazing. His name was Doctor Payne, and he was the head sinus surgeon at that teaching hospital, University of Virginia Medical Center in Charlottesville. (We thought that was a rather unfortunate name for a surgeon. lol. You would think if your last name was "pain," medicine would not be the field you'd choose. I'd play football or something. But I'm sure glad he became a sinus surgeon! He was a skilled doctor, the top dude in the area.)

The difference in how I felt was amazing. When something happens so gradually over many years, you don't really notice how lousy you're feeling. (And investigation showed that my sinus issues started when I was hit in the head with a sledge hammer roughly fourteen years earlier! And no, Sheila didn't hit me.) When the discomfort finally comes to a head, and then the problem is solved, the difference is so drastic! I thought, "How in the world did I ever live before?"

But again, a spiritual parallel. That's what the world does—just gradually, gradually, gradually piles on more and more stuff, like the frog in the boiling water. You just don't notice it. Until finally you turn to Jesus and He removes it. You think, "My gosh, how did I ever cope before?" God is showing me through this whole process—while I was going through it and now that I'm looking back—so much of the physical has a spiritual lesson. Physical circumstances are so often a mirror or a shadow of what we are dealing with spiritually. We can learn from everything that happens.

January 29, 2015 Evening
Game on…Sheila's two hands wrestling the phone out of Brian's left hand…success! But it took quite a lot of effort! Yeah!

February 2, 2015

Brian continues to feel great and **so** improved after the sinus surgery last Wednesday! I've heard him comment to many people how his entire body feels better! He can't get over what an immediate difference the surgery made. I guess it makes sense that if you had such a deep-seated infection that had been there and growing for years—that close to your brain—yes, thank you, Lord! I'm hoping he'll do a video update later this morning. Thanks everyone for your prayers!

He can sing again now after the sinus surgery! Yeah! We thought it was just the stroke effects that were keeping him from singing. And the guitar playing is definitely getting better, quicker changes and more agility! Go, God!

I recorded him playing guitar and singing in the studio here. Amazing improvement! He really couldn't sing before the sinus surgery. Thank you, Lord!

February 5, 2015

Have I mentioned lately how much I love this young man? He has a tender heart toward the Lord and others, loves his family, and has a quiet strength. These last seven months have not been easy on him—seeing his dad, who has always been the strong one, struggling to regain his health. Colton stepped up immediately, understanding and taking it seriously that he was the "man of the house" for five weeks while Brian was in the hospital. He is a joy to be around 98 percent of the time, which is quite a statement to make of 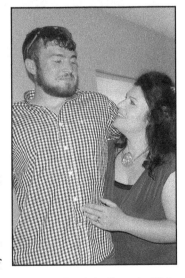 any teenager! In a couple weeks he will turn twenty! Can't believe it. This momma sure is proud and grateful. Love you, Son.

February 7, 2015

Blessings this past week: $200 from someone who didn't want Pampered Chef but wanted to contribute, meat from a friend, a case of paper towels and bottled water. Three new piano students this past month. Taxes done … refunds coming.

February 8, 2015

Pray about sinus appointment tomorrow at UVA at 11:00 AM. Still feels much improved but stuffy on the left side now. Hope we get clearance for a cross-country trip to Texas, too!

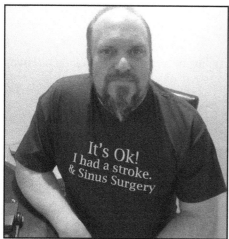 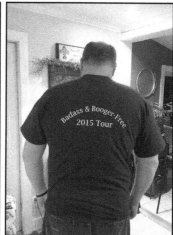

February 9, 2015

Home from UVA sinus surgery check up … prayed for a total stranger in the restroom who was obviously in a lot of pain, watched the range of sunshine to cloudy to rain on Afton mountain, made the doctor laugh by seeing Brian's new T-shirt.

"It's OK! I had a stroke and sinus surgery." On the back it says, "Badass and Booger-Free Tour 2016."

The doctor even took pictures and asked if he could post them on his Facebook wall. lol

Doctor's findings upon inspection (roughly 12-inch-long metal camera scope eased up into the high reaches of Brian's sinuses!—Yikes!) says there is still a lot of inflammation and some infection on both the right and left sides. So he switched up antibiotics, cleaned him out really well (**Yuck**—I watched the screen), and scheduled a recheck in four weeks.

He **cleared** us to travel on our trip across country to Texas next week! Yeah! ... more about that in a few days. Thanks for the prayers.

As I drove the 100 or so miles over to UVA this morning, I found that my mind was busily running through plans, to-do lists, how to juggle $ to cover the bills and similar details. With worship music on in the background (don't underestimate the importance of what we allow into our hearing)... I stopped and asked myself a question that I asked quite often at the beginning of this journey, "Lord, what is it You are wanting to be to me right now that you could not be any other time?"

The answer I sensed was about **daily bread**. Jesus taught His disciples to pray, and one of the specific lines was, "Give us this day our daily bread." We say we need to take things one day at a time but truly that is not easy to do. However, through this journey, the Lord has never once failed to meet one of our needs. And He never will, because being a Provider is part of His character.

I sensed this morning that He just wanted to say, "Sheila, it's a beautiful day for a drive in this gorgeous part of the country that is your home right now. Enjoy the scenery. Enjoy the fact that your husband continues to make excellent progress. Trust me that I am making in him full restoration, full healing—body, soul, mind, and spirit. Enjoy the time together. You have a full tank of gas, a nice car to drive, money for lunch, and a good doctor addressing his needs. As far as the future, I've got it. Don't worry about tomorrow. Tomorrow will worry about itself. Each day has enough trouble of its own... and this is a good day."

Amen.

LESSON: REST IN THE LORD

February 9, 2015 BRIAN: REST in the Lord

Driving over to UVA for a checkup after the first sinus surgery. I remember it was a beautiful day—nice temperature, everything. The sun was shining, and Sheila was driving so I was able to sit in the car and think. I was talking to God as we were driving, praying, and I remember that's the first time in this journey that I felt the idea of "**rest** in Him" coming to my mind. I had been so focused on recovery, regaining strength, getting "back to myself" and all this other stuff that everyone was expecting me to "get back to"—which I wanted as well! I always felt God's peace through the whole ordeal, but this was the first time I really grasped this idea of real rest.

The truth was that no matter what happens, I can rest in Christ. Really rest. Not just abide. Not just shelter myself, but I can truly rest in Him. And that quality is what brings lasting peace, contentment with Jesus—enjoying the beautiful day, the birds chirping, the sun coming over the hills, feeling the rays warm my face. I was astounded at the beauty that He has created, along with the realization of how much better it's going to be with everything renewed! This world has been decaying since Adam, for how many thousands of years, and it's still an astonishingly beautiful place.

Yes, I think that day was the first I was aware of His rest in such a deep way. God has continued throughout this process of recovery (almost three years into it at this writing) to show me more and more…but we'll get into that later. I just remember that day being the first time I truly felt that idea of rest in a way that I hadn't been taught or hadn't thought of…ever. I was under the mindset of "You don't rest. You work!"

Sheila: Well, in that mindset, one is trying to provide for him/herself.

Brian: Yes, and you're trying to get more, do better, be successful. You're working so hard to try to find that place of contentment. And for me, that was ever so elusive! The moment I thought I had it, the target would move.

Sheila: It's ironic that we work hard to try to find contentment, but we do.

Brian: I always thought, "Well, I'm going to work hard to gain everything I can get. Then there will come a point when I can just stop and enjoy what I've done." I don't know why I had that mindset in my head, but that's just our culture's philosophy. The world doesn't provide contentment or rest. You might "make it" financially, but if you are successful in that realm, then there's something else nagging at you, something that is just out of your reach. You think, "Oh, if I could just get _____, I'd be happy. Then I could rest and just enjoy, maintain." It doesn't work that way in the world. But it **does** in Christ! I can rest in knowing Christ, knowing that He has saved me; He provides for me. He'll continue to provide. He might have work for me to do—and Scripture says that He sets up work in advance for us to do (Ephesians 2:10 NIV). However, I don't work to achieve that contentment, peace, and rest. Those qualities come with Christ. And they're free.

We got home to notices in the mailbox which require administrative attention, the Expedition won't start, piano students coming shortly, Colton trying to sort out a confusing letter from DMV, and Brian being fairly worn out from the excavating that occurred deep in his sinuses a few hours ago.

DAILY BREAD. Daily provision. Thank you, Lord.
And as far as tomorrow is concerned, God is already there. We can rest in Him.

February 10, 2015
We had to buy a new starter for the truck … $137. I dug through a few years of receipts trying to find the original because it has a lifetime warranty. Found one, just not sure it's the right one so we'll see tomorrow. **But** regardless, there was a donation that came in today on the WeCaring site for $97. Thanks, Lord.

Seven months today.

Seven is God's number of perfection or completion. Yes, Lord!

Where are we today? Well, Brian is outside with his dad fixing the starter on the Expedition in the cold. For the last nearly 3 hours I have been sitting at my kitchen table doing a variety of administrative tasks—writing a letter to a congressman (a friend works for him and recommended we do it), requesting help with some things. Texting back and forth with Aimee Patrick trying to clear up deductibles, etc., with Anthem. (She is faster than Google!) Sorting through info for the kids while we are on our trip to Texas, leaving next week.

But here's good news! We got a letter from DDS yesterday scheduling an appointment for Brian with a medical examiner. This is more information needed by Disability. The initial appointment was made for when we are still out of state. Brian called and spoke to a very kind, helpful government worker who was glad to change the appointment. So … it's March 17th. Please pray for God's perfect plan in this.

Check up this afternoon with our local family doctor and staff. It's always a pleasure seeing them!

Brian notices improvement in his sinuses since the medicine change yesterday. Thank God! We are praying that the infection gets all cleared **out** of his body.

Thanks for your continued prayers. Please continue to pray for him to remain encouraged. Even though he is able to do some things, he cannot do them at the level to which he is used to. That gets frustrating and discouraging at times… even when he knows all the "right spiritual answers."

February 11, 2015

Spiritual attack this morning. I just felt D O N E. Reached out for prayer and bound the enemy in the name of **Jesus**. Then I meditated on Matthew 11:28–30 NIV. Jesus said, *"Come to me you who are weary and burdened, and I will give you rest. Take my yoke upon you and learn from me for I am gentle and humble in heart, and you will find rest for your souls. For my yoke is easy and my burden is light."*

1 Peter 1:7 NIV: *"These (all kinds of trials) have come … so that your faith – of greater worth than gold which perishes even though refined by fire – may be proved genuine and may result in praise, glory and honor when Jesus Christ is revealed."*

February 12, 2015

Received some great encouragement today from a visit with a dear friend. Thanks, Robby Meadows, for coming over to hang out with us this morning!

For the last 24 hours I've had Garrett with diarrhea (and he never has had much of a concept of making it to the toilet… I won't go into more detail than that), Brian in bad pain from pulling a muscle (I guess) in his right shoulder. Appreciate prayers. At least G will get this bug out of his system before we leave Monday.

We're rounding out the night with a visit from a friend who had been trying to connect for a while. Thank you, Lord, for a great time of fellowship, mutual encouragement, worship, and prayer together! We have such a treasure in the Body of Christ. May we make the effort and take the time required to nurture and develop those relationships.

February 13, 2015

I am working ahead in my homework for the "Believing God" (by Beth Moore) ladies' Bible study. I'm watching session three talking about believing that God can do what He says He can do. She makes a profound statement based on Mark 9:23 NIV, *"Everything is possible for one who believes."* Sadly, most of us are caught in a cycle of unbelief. In other words, we believe little because we have seen little, and we've seen little because we believe little. Oh, Lord, help us to believe big!

Throughout this journey with Brian's recovery, many people have commented, "You guys have such great faith." Although we appreciate the encouragement, please know that the same faith is available to everyone who believes in Jesus Christ! Faith is a gift from God to all who ask. It is also a muscle: the more we exercise it, the stronger it gets. But it's based on believing that God is who He says He is and that He can do what He says He can do!

I'm not talking about sensationalism, where we are consumed by looking for miracles. I'm talking about believing what the Bible says and walking it out in our day-to-day life. Will you join me?

February 14, 2015

Interesting how God changes my perspective. Spent a little bit of time this afternoon with several of us from church baptizing an elderly lady in a nursing home. Several of us crowded into her room—TV on, baby running around—down-to-earth, real life infused with the Spirit of Christ and the sacrament of baptism done with no fanfare or flourish. It reminded me that Jesus is willing to come in anywhere at anytime. He just needs an invitation.

It wasn't lost on me that not long ago Brian and I were spending an awful lot of time in a rehab facility/hospital. Our lives usually just go on and we don't think about the people who are struggling. I pray peace for them today in Jesus' name.

February 15, 2015

Tomorrow Brian and I will be setting out on a drive across country to Fort Davis, Texas. It is in the far southwest corner of the state, very close to the border of Mexico! We have a few friends there who are in ministry, and we've felt a draw to investigate our potential involvement. Our first trip was August 2013. But on a broader scale, we have sensed for quite some time (over two years so long before the stroke) that the Lord was preparing us to make a leap of faith, dive into a new season and new way of life. Obviously, the stroke has brought about such an opportunity, but we do still feel a pull to move West. This trip will allow us the time and rest to contemplate and pray.

We are looking forward to a couple weeks of respite as well as some warmer climates! It's 59 degrees there right now and headed to the 70s in a couple days! Please keep us in prayer for God's perfect plan for this time.

The boys are staying home. Feel free to check in on them and offer them food. Lol

TRIP ACROSS COUNTRY TO FORT DAVIS, TEXAS

February 16, 2015

I had forgotten until Brian prayed at the start of our trip this morning that God laid this trip on his heart while he was still in rehab back in July—that once he was doing better and could drive, we would take an extended trip across country to seek His plan for the future and also just to enjoy. Amen! Thanks, Lord, for the time, ability, and provision.

Was harder than I expected leaving the kids. We're on the road.... Left around 8:40 AM. Late start because neither of us moved off the couch yesterday. I was sick, and his shoulder pain has been bad. I felt lousy, so of course couldn't do all the things you normally do the day before a trip to get ready. Going to bed that night I prayed, "OK, Father, if you want us to take this trip, You have to let us feel better in the morning. Or we're simply not going to be able to leave. The big snowstorm is coming heavy on our tail too. If we don't leave tomorrow morning, we'll be snowed in for a few days. So it's up to You. I put it in Your hands."

We both slept well and felt good in the morning.

*** *Looking back afterwards, we truly believe our various illnesses had been a spiritual attack attempting to keep us from going. God had so much in store for us on that trip in so many ways! The enemy did not want that to happen. It was a time of incredible refreshment just for the two of* *us. Such a needed change after everything we've been through! And we were sincerely seeking God's will for our future.*

Love to all. Thanks for prayers. Ten-hour drive today to Jackson, TN. Finished lunch in Fort Chiswell, Virginia. Chatted with cashier at gas station. She's been a caregiver for a while... her grandmother then her husband dealing with cancer, surgery, etc. I can relate to the caregiver now! We talked about the strength the Lord provides. Her husband is now cancer-free!

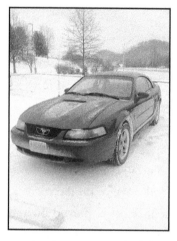

Not the best winter storm traveling vehicle. So be it.

February 17, 2015

We would've been on the road earlier this morning, but I got chatting with a couple during the continental breakfast at the hotel. Talked to husband while she ate. He was standing with their dog, Lucy. Had been in WWII and is eighty-eight years old. Wife's name was Evelyn and he told me they'd been married sixty-four years—said she was three at the time! They were delightful. No children—she said they stay together because they like each other! We discussed one another's trips and she said, "I'll pray for you, kid!"

February 18, 2015

Mississippi! We got an early start today... partly due to sleeping in a hotel room less than a football field from a busy highway, loud snoring, and sharing a double bed with my king-size husband. So... I was up a little after 4:00 AM, and we were on the road at 6:00 AM! Ugh. **Not** this girl's favorite time zone, lol. Nothing but sunshine rising temperatures from here on out. Destination today: Dallas/Fort Worth at least.

February 19, 2015

We are in a gorgeous hotel room, and I am doing some Bible study.

Look at Colossians 1:15–18 NIV

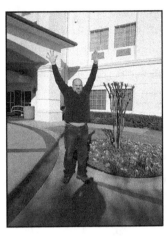

The Son is the image of the invisible God, the firstborn over all creation. For in him all things were created: things in heaven and on earth, visible and invisible, whether thrones or powers or rulers or authorities; all things have been created through him and for him. He is before all things, and in him all things hold together. And he is the head of the body, the church; he is the beginning and the firstborn from among the dead, so that in everything he might have the supremacy.

It's all about Jesus! He was not just a good man or wonderful teacher/prophet. He was and is the Son of God!

FEB 15, 2015

Brian: Trip to Texas and warmth of the sun

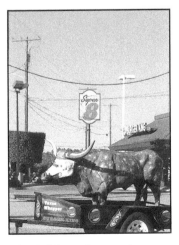

On our trip to Texas, I remember stopping at a hotel just after we'd crossed into Texas. I realized that the warmth, the heat of the sun, made a difference to my body. The winter back home would tighten my left side up, and it would get harder to move. Whereas on the trip as we would get to warmer and warmer climates, I could feel things loosening up, and I could move better. I'm not saying it was 100 percent better, but noticeably better.

Once again I think that's a parallel of a spiritual condition—when we are in the Light and the warmth of Christ, we move around better. We are more limber. When we get in the cold or the darkness, away from Christ and God, we tighten up. We tend to close up. It's as if we go into a protective mode because we are looking to our own strength, which is inadequate compared to Christ.

Our stop for the night... Weatherford, Texas. Not really far today, but still a good day. Had the windows down much of the afternoon! What temperature is it at home again? You think that's pretty mean, but come on... he **did** have a **stroke** and sinus surgery! Give him a break. Lol

February 20, 2015

I say on my FB wall, "It's 74!"

My cousin from western Pennsylvania posts that there's a 77-degree difference!

After hours of flat plains on I-20W, we get on the "Rabbit Road" (2903) heading towards Fort Davis. Absolutely breathtaking...

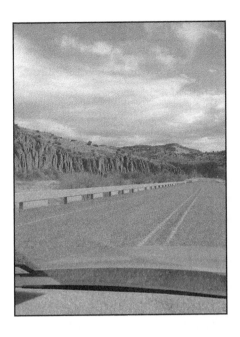

February 21, 2015

Some guerrilla worship and prayer today. (Guerrilla Worship is something God laid on Brian's heart a few years ago. It involves praying over the land, singing and/or playing praises to the Lord, and declaring the reign of Jesus in every way.)

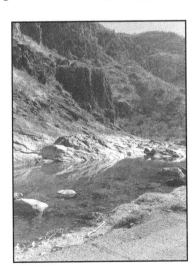
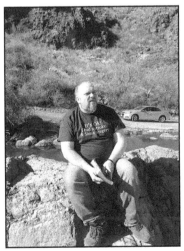

February 22, 20015

Just to let all of our northern snow bunnies know ... we are experiencing a cold front today. It is raining with a low of 27 degrees tonight. Needed gas. Pumps in town let you use a card even though the station is closed. Then we drove 24 miles (through beautiful mountain scenes but virtually no signs of civilization) to the nearest town to fill up the tank. Interesting.

*** *It took me quite a while of living out here to realize that all of that open land with no signs of civilization is privately owned ranch land. The space is just so different from back East! Land is divided into "sections," which consist of 640 acres. Ranches are made of x number of sections—it is poor etiquette to ask how large someone's ranch is or how many cattle they have. That would be like asking someone how much money they have in the bank! I did spend time on one private ranch which had been written up in Texas Monthly, therefore it had been publicized it consisted of over 50,000 acres! One could drive for hours and never leave their land! I also learned that because of the high desert climate, to effectively raise one cow, roughly 62 acres is needed. No wonder the ranches are so big. Interestingly, though, the grasses the Lord causes to grow here, although sparse by eastern definition, contain much more minerals and proteins per capita.*

Literally, you can drive for hours out here and see only open land. It is an amazing reality and one that really has become soothing to me rather than stifling or frustrating. (Although, I admit it gets old having to drive 3 hours to the airport or over an hour to the nearest Walmart/shopping mall/ chain restaurant such as Garrett's all-time favorite, AppleBees. However, the long car rides become excellent opportunities for true conversations, rich fellowship or alone time with the Lord—often without any cell service or internet to disrupt the flow. Brian and I have spent countless hours together in the car, whether driving just to nearby Alpine 24 miles away or 2 hours one way to see a medical specialist, or all the way to Houston —which is 10 hours one way—for the checkups with the neuro therapist. God has used the time to de-stress, reconnect us, or give us opportunity to discuss and discern His leading.) The remote aspects of living here have been a main contributor of rest and unplugging from the rat race of the world—which is an agreed-upon benefit according to nearly every person we have encountered, whether full-time resident or vacationer.

February 24, 2015
I neglected to mention that we enjoyed such a special evening Sunday at house church. The Lord had some specific words of encouragement for us personally, and the time of worship was awesome.

*** We met Jim and Judy Spradley for the first time, who became dear friends as well as mentors/encouragers in the faith to us. The Lord used them—and continues to do so—in many ways.

February 26, 2015 would have been Dad's ninety-ninth birthday
Yesterday we drove down to Big Bend National Park (Southwest Texas) and spent several hours driving through a small portion of it. I don't think I have ever seen any sights so amazing! Glory to God!

We ended yesterday by sitting in the home of new friends, talking about what God has been doing in our lives and hearing their stories as well. There couldn't have been a better way to end the day! Made me think of Malachi 3:16.

Malachi 3:16 NIV: "Then those who feared the Lord talked with each other, and the Lord listened and heard. A scroll of remembrance was written in his presence concerning those who feared the Lord and honored his name."

I know I have posted mostly pix and fun things, but we are hearing **lots** from the Lord on this trip, so we thank you for your prayers. Keep 'em coming!

The Rio Grand.... As soon as your feet touch the riverbed, you are in Mexico. Brian was determined to walk through rough terrain and over rocks in the riverbed to put his hand in the water. We all prayed together too. Was a really special time. Seven-and-a-half months ago he had a stroke, and today he did all this with no cane and no foot brace! It was not easy but he did it! Thank you, Lord!

February 27, 2015

We have been reminded here about how the Lord works "behind the scenes" often for years or even decades, but then "suddenly" something comes to pass. We think that just because we aren't seeing things God is not at work. But God is always at work!

February 28, 2015

It's gorgeous and sunny today, around 60 degrees. I took a long walk through town.

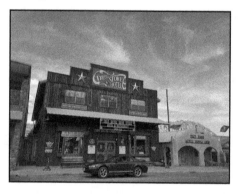

More about our trip to Texas: February 16–March 7, 2015. Even the process of getting out the door was under spiritual warfare. Brian's right shoulder pain, my sickness, the snowstorm and ice. We were both truly exhausted and in no physical condition to the naked eye to make a big trip. I prayed the night before, "OK, Lord, if you want me to go you have to give me strength." And He did. We left the next morning. We knew we needed to leave. It was a matter of obedience and looking back, probably very prophetic.

* We arrived Friday, February 20, in Fort Davis and were blessed with the "Arabella" studio to stay in. It was private, comfortable, and exactly what we needed. There was renewal in every area—intimacy, rest, peace. Meals were provided. It was a wonderful vacation!

*   On February 21, Colton's 20th birthday, Brian sensed the need for our friends to pray for him in the mountains. So we did, near the Boy Scout camp.
*   House church on the 22nd … God spoke many words strongly through Jim Spradley, including "Get in the boat and go to the other side. Speak to the left side, wake up in Jesus' name!" Jim also said, "You have waited on the persistence of Jesus." It went through me like a knife spiritually each time he said it.
*   On the 23rd I did artwork along with a couple friends. With my painting I felt like God blessed me by teaching me how to do it and allowing beauty to come forth.
*   On the 24th Brian and I sat at The Drugstore (The iconic restaurant in the center of town owned by our friends) sharing what God is doing, hearing the vision the Lord is giving for Fort Davis. We prayerfully wondered how God would have us be involved.
*   On Wednesday the 25th we went to Big Bend National Park—wow! The greatness of God! Brian made the effort to walk down the path to the Rio Grande.

    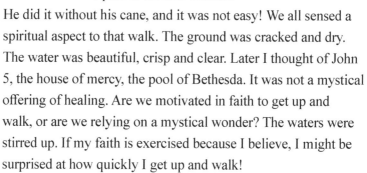

    He did it without his cane, and it was not easy! We all sensed a spiritual aspect to that walk. The ground was cracked and dry. The water was beautiful, crisp and clear. Later I thought of John 5, the house of mercy, the pool of Bethesda. It was not a mystical offering of healing. Are we motivated in faith to get up and walk, or are we relying on a mystical wonder? The waters were stirred up. If my faith is exercised because I believe, I might be surprised at how quickly I get up and walk!
*   In the evening we spent time at a friend's home. Was a rich time of fellowship, sharing stories and prayer.
*   Several other experiences and connections while we were there, all of which served to deepen our sense of call to the area.

BACK HOME ... LESSONS FROM THE TRIP

BRIAN: about the trip to Fort Davis, Texas, in February 2015

I've been thinking about how we took the trip to Texas even though people thought we were crazy. I'm sure many thought, "What are you doing taking a big trip like that—using all that money for something not necessary? You're not strong enough. You're going to drive across country...?" But we just felt like we were supposed to go.

God taught us several lessons:

"You're stronger than you think. In Christ you're able to do the trip." The trip was not a hardship on me physically. I was able to drive majority of the time, even in the snow. Even funnier was that we were in the Mustang—which I thought was hilarious—passing all the four-wheel drive trucks stuck in the median, while we motored along in our 2002 Mustang. God's hand was on us! Getting out to the West—to the warmth, the heat— in the middle of winter was significant. Going to the Rio Grande in Big Bend National Park was significant—walking down to the river without a cane was incredibly hard on my left leg, but I was able to do it. God just kept saying, "Take another step. Just take another step. Don't quit.

Take another step." And before you knew it, I was there and back. I wasn't expecting to dip my hand in the water and be completely healed; that wasn't what I was hearing in my spirit. God was showing me, "You can do it when you trust in me. Focus on Me, not on the length of the walk. But focus on My voice. Focus on My face. Focus on My words." And before I know it, I was there. That was the lesson.

Then we learned something else. Somebody we had met handed us a check, a big check, that covered almost all of the trip. A couple other people gave us cash donations as well because they wanted to bless us. What we thought or others thought was a waste of money—How can we afford to go on a trip like this when I'm not working and Sheila is giving up three weeks of piano lessons, and Disability money had not come through yet...?—But we did it because we believed we had heard God say, "Go." So we went, and God provided a way that paid for the trip and made up the deficit. That was a lesson learned.

When you follow God—not that you're going to get rich, that's not what I'm saying—but when you follow the Lord, He takes care of things. It doesn't have to make sense in the world's eyes. In fact, it rarely does. It just has to be what God is saying to do. And you obey without question. You do it with your understanding of the Word realizing that God is not going to tell you to do one thing one time and contradict Himself another time. He's not going to go against His own Word. We need to be like the Bereans in Acts 17:11—if you have the Word in your head, you will know whether something is lining up or not.

Sometimes it might not be God whom you're hearing. But in this case, it was. And we learned big lessons for which we were thankful, grateful, and joyful.

It was a great trip even though I was still pretty weak. He showed me that He's never left me. He's still there, and He always will be.

March 1, 2015

Got this quote from a friend at the perfect time. Even though we believe and see that God is healing Brian ... back to full restoration, better than new ... sometimes it is difficult because it is not completed yet. The process gets old some days.

Our friend said, "I appreciated this quote from an article in *Charisma Magazine* called When God Delays the Answer to Your Prayer. I thought of you as you continue to wait.

"God designed what we perceive a delay as an opportunity to not only answer our prayer, but to give us more than we asked for."

Match 9, 2015

Just want to say thank you to those of you who prayed for us during our trip to Texas and back. What an adventure! I think we did a total of about 3,500 miles, certainly taking the scenic route and avoiding the winter storms when we could. One really interesting aspect was seeing how the land changes throughout the various states. On the way out, we went through Virginia, West Virginia, Tennessee, Alabama, Louisiana, Mississippi and pretty much all the way across Texas, as Fort Davis is in the lower SW corner. Then coming home we went back across Texas (but on I-10 not I-20 this time), across Louisiana, Mississippi, Alabama, then Georgia, South Carolina, North Carolina, and finally Virginia.

Driving across country has been a long time dream for Brian. His ideal would be to do it in an old car and on only secondary roads rather than interstate. I, however, am thankful we had a newer car and followed mainly interstates. But it was really a step of faith for us to take the trip. Obviously, mine is the only income right now; taking three weeks off from teaching was significant. We believed the Lord wanted us to do it, so we did. During the trip, we were given a generous monetary gift, which pretty much made up the deficit. God is so good!

We had requested prayer for rest, rejuvenation, refreshment, and also some clarity as to the next steps of where the Lord wants us in ministry. He answered on all fronts, and more richly than we could imagine.

Brian has a checkup with sinus doctor at UVA today. Last time he still had a lot of infection. Hope that it is cleared up now.

$$ issues ... Virginia Heart Associates approved our financial aid, so $0 balance there. Fairfax Radiology denied it, and the $1,038 balance remains.

BUT big news ... Anthem finally approved the helicopter ride! Thank you, Jesus!!

Brian has a medical exam with the Disability people next Tuesday ... appreciate prayers.

*** *Looking back I realize once again how significant that trip to Texas was! Since the summer of 2012 we had felt called to move to Fort Davis, Texas. We were very close to putting our house on the market when the stroke hit. With the stroke drastically changing every aspect of our lives, we needed to know if the Lord was still calling us to move. That trip was a fleece. But we did not realize at the time how much we needed a change of perspective, a vacation and a time of rest. We left our home not even knowing where we would stay in Texas, which was actually very pro-phetic, as we basically repeated that when we actually moved. We were offered a beautiful place to stay and were graciously provided for during our visit in meals as well as fellowship, which again was echoed when we actually moved. It was refreshing not only to be in the warm climate, but also to see a completely different culture and landscape. I have learned in my life—through Garrett's birth as well as this experience—sometimes in order to walk a new path you have to be able to see differently, be in new surroundings. The desert climate was well suited for us at that time. We did not come to understand that fully until a couple years later. God knew. The trip was a huge blessing and a real time of refreshment. But then we arrived back home and had to jump right back in to the reality of life, doctors, therapy, recovery....*

MORE RECOVERY AND
DEALING WITH DEBT

March 11, 2015

The sinus culture the doctor took Monday still shows infection, so Brian will do another round of antibiotics plus some ointments in his sinus rinse (yeah, fun stuff!). He said, "Guess we really just didn't realize how bad those sinuses were!"

But he was encouraged yesterday when he stopped in to see some friends and they commented how much better he looked and was getting around since they had seen him! Yay!

Yesterday was eight months since the stroke. Biblically, the number 8 signifies new beginnings. Yes, Lord! We will accept that in Jesus' name.

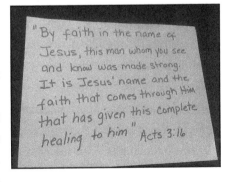

A mystery encourager left this in my car before sunrise one morning back a few months ago. It has been in view in our kitchen ever since. Lord, **I still believe** you said full healing and full restoration.

I don't say that as a pie in the sky or a Pollyanna attitude. I truly believe the Lord spoke that to my heart within the first few hours of the stroke.

Doing my bible study this morning, I was reminded of the fact that often the promises of God took a loonnnnngggg time to come to pass. For example, God promised Abraham that his descendants would receive the promised land. But check out Genesis 15:12–18 and Acts 7:17 and Hebrews 11:22. Notice how long that promise was in process before fulfillment—well over 400 years!

I appreciated that reminder today as sometimes we (especially Brian) get weary of the process and frustrated with his limitations. But then I am reminded in simple ways how **much** better he is! For example, walking up the steps to our friends' home Monday night which is steep and with no railing— in August he couldn't do it at all; then needed a lot of help by people in front and beside and his four-prong cane; then could do it with a little help and four-prong cane; little help and walking stick; minimal help and no walking stick ... then Monday night going up practically on his own. It is in those moments I am reminded of the process and so grateful for the improvements!

March 14, 2015 PUBLIC JOURNAL

Yesterday was a tough day, full of mixed emotions. It began in the morning with both Brian and I spending a lot of time on the phone dealing with creditors and exploring options. After being out of work for eight months, things really get tight **and yet** we are constantly reminded of God's provision for all of our needs and even many of our wants! (I mean, look, we took a three-week trip across the country!)

But we were no longer able to make the credit card payments (of around $400/month) as of February, so the calls and letters started to come in. We also have a couple medical bills from places that have not offered financial aid. Visa referred us to a debt counselor, but after taking our debt-income ratio, she was unable to offer us any viable options besides bankruptcy.

When you are laying out the facts financially on paper, it looks rather bleak **humanly** speaking. I had to repeat myself so many times and I ended up in tears more than once—again with total strangers on the phone! I figure there might have been purpose in it, and indeed I did speak with a couple people who really acted like human beings and seemed to have compassion.

Anyway, the rest of the day we both struggled with discouragement and had to fight off worry and fear financially more than we ever have had in this whole journey. I realized too that **shame** was trying to lay ahold of me for making those poor financial decisions years ago in the first place. So I had to pray and remind the enemy that I have repented, been forgiven, **and** that the Lord has mercifully removed the ramifications from the past! Romans 8:1 NIV, *"There is therefore now **no** condemnation for those who are in Christ Jesus!"*

When Brian and I were talking about it later in the day and this morning, he said, "You know, we all owed a debt we could not pay. Jesus came and paid it for us! This whole thing is a great parallel and reminder of redemption!"

Credit card debt is a great example because it is so unwise, and those mistakes from the past follow you for years and years. You can't ever seem to break free of them. Just like in our lives, the enemy wants to remind us of our sin and make us feel foolish. However, Jesus took all the blame, all the shame, all the consequences! He paid the debt we could never pay and gave us an opportunity to return to a complete and whole relationship with a loving Father. It is a **free** gift; we just need to say 'Yes!"

And so I say, "Thank you, Lord, for this reminder, this very graphic but clear representation of redemption. And I thank you that You are not only our Redeemer but You are our Provider. You know every need. You have always been faithful and You will continue to be because that is Your very nature. Faithfulness is inherent in Your very character, as is Mercy, Grace, Love, Peace. Thank You, Jesus!"

March 14, 2015 later
I forgot a very important part of my earlier post (that started with "day of mixed emotions")...

In the midst of those frustrating phone calls, my cell phone rang. It was one of my closest friends, but I couldn't talk right then. I let it go to voicemail. A couple hours later I finally wrapped up the phone calls and listened to her voicemail. She said that during her quiet time, the Spirit had laid a phrase of scripture on her heart and pressed upon her that she was to call me and tell me to **write** it down.

Now, this is not a friend who normally has these kinds of promptings … which, frankly, made me take notice all the more.

Stunned, I replayed the message three times. I knew immediately the scripture reference because it is one that the Lord has brought to me a few times over the last several years. It is not a common scripture to come across, but there have been three specific times that this verse has come to me. Each time it is a glaring reminder of God's eye on me and an assurance of His calling.

What a sweet reminder! In the midst of such frustration, it was as if the Lord was saying to me, "Daughter, I see you. I'm here. My plan is still in effect."

Thank you, Lord.

BRIAN: credit card debts and how God got us debt-free
It's kind of funny that throughout the whole stroke process—almost eight months in—I haven't worked and Disability hadn't come through, so we've been living on Sheila's income and donations. But up until that point, we had not missed a payment. We did make a few proactive calls to a couple creditors explaining the situation and asking if any accommodations could be made. We asked if there were any provisions to see if we could reduce things for a while, but there was nothing available.

At first I was kind of angry at God. I thought, "You know, God, we had finally gotten to the point where we were starting to get ahead a little bit." Our kids were grown. Colton had a job, was getting out on his own, taking care of his own bills. We were finally able to save again. We figured in a few months or year or two, we'd be doing a lot better. We were feeling that breathing room which many couples experience when their kids are grown—when you don't have that expense anymore. (We did have Garrett, but Garrett is really fairly easy.) And that's when the stroke happened.

So, yes, I was a little angry at God at that point. I'd say, "Lord, we just can't catch a break! Really, now I have a stroke?!" God reminded me that I had to swallow my pride, which is not easy for a man to do I think, and call the credit card company to say, "Here's what happened. I've been out of work since July of 2014. Up until now we've been able to keep everything current, but starting next month, it's not going to be. Because we just can't. The little pile of money we had has gradually dwindled down to where we can pay the mortgage, keep the lights on, gas in the tank, and have food on the table but unfortunately, making your credit card payment is not a bare necessity. I don't mean to say that cruelly or spitefully; it's just the facts."

The lady understood, but she couldn't understand why I was calling. She kept saying, "Wait. Your account's in good standing. You're calling to tell me you're **going** to be delinquent on your payment—not why you **are** but that you're going to be?!" She had never had anyone do that before. While I was talking to her, it hit me: Jesus reminded me that in the humbling of myself to call and talk to these companies is the parallel of redemption.

We only had two credit cards, and some might say we didn't have as much debt as many Americans, but it was too much. It was that nagging bill—as soon as we'd start to get ahead, something else went wrong requiring another purchase. (Obviously, we had gotten to the place that we did not have ample breathing room in our budget, which of course is not wise.)

Christ reminded me that in the humbling of myself, we all owe a debt we cannot pay at some point. Christ Jesus pays the debt for us. It's like He said, "If you will humble yourself and take this on, explain to them what's going on, then I will work in the situation.

Humble yourself. Tell the truth. Share the facts. Don't try to make anything of it that it isn't and I'll take care of it." God will take care of it. You know, it's funny, within a fairly short time—I'm sure Sheila will have the exact details in her journals!— God really changed our financial situation.

One time Sheila was on the phone with a credit card company and asked, "Will you take a cash settlement right now to forgive this debt?" They negotiated down and basically took between 30–40 cents on the dollar. I thought, "Well, okay, where am I going to come up with that money?" Then I remembered a life insurance policy that an agent had kind of talked me into buying early in our marriage. I didn't even have to take away from the benefit amount; I had some cash value built up. I was able to withdraw it under no penalty. I even asked the life insurance agent, "I can take x amount of money and turn it into x amount of money paying off some debt." She said, "That's always a smart move! I'll get you that money asap."

So basically within a week we had enough money to settle the debt on both of those credit cards from that insurance policy as well as a tax return. (The second one wasn't resolved for a few more months—more about that later.) We were able to pay those credit cards off for pennies on the dollar.

It was amazing how God moved! In a short period of time we finally came to the bottom of ourselves with the debt situation. We had to swallow our pride, call them. Then the Lord worked it all out: we got the insurance money, our tax refund in the mail, and the notice that Disability had come through. We also got a letter from the IRS saying that they had made a mistake on our taxes, and we were owed a large additional refund.

It's like in the course of a few days, God said, "Look, just don't give in to despair. Don't give in to lack of hope. Don't give in to fear. I can change things on a dime any way I want to!" We went from thinking we might have to let the house go, or just not knowing how we were going to be able to make the finances work long term, feeling like some of this stuff was beginning to overwhelm us. We went from that to the promise of several thousand between Disability and what the IRS was saying.

I didn't know if it was actually going to work out like that or not, but nevertheless God made His point. He said, "Don't despair. I can always show you hope. There is always hope in Me." It was a moment of rejoicing and crying. I remember Sheila and I holding each other in the car looking at the letter that came in the mail, being in awe and dumbfounded at the grace of God.

Only in the valleys do you really see God work that way. If you don't go through hardships, if you never face troubles, if you don't go through persecution, you don't always see that. I think that's the point of why God lets us go through suffering and hard times— so that we can see His grace. We can see His mercy. We can see His love; we can recognize it and be thankful for it.

March 14, 2015
Brian resumed his OT yesterday after being gone. Expert therapist Amy Gray tested his grip strength. The first day of therapy back in August it was 15 pounds of pressure for his left hand. Yesterday it was 50 pounds, consistently three times! The right hand has increased too—from 100 pounds to 120 pounds. Wow! She was thrilled. She also did the light meter test, which is a huge board that covers the wall and tiny squares light up randomly. He has to touch each square as quickly as possible. His reactions had greatly improved in that as well.

Then she shared something with us from the notes of the first session about his having an "Asymmetric Tonic Neck Reflex." She said she would never have told us this at the beginning but she could tell us now … ATNR means that when Brian lifted his left arm, he turned his head in the opposite direction. This is contrary to a normal motion and is usually indicative of a poor recovery/restoration. Well, praise God that has **not** been the case! Once again, thank you, Jesus!

DISABILITY EXAM

March 17, 2015 PUBLIC JOURNAL
Disability medical exam today at 1:30. Appreciate prayers.

March 17, 2015 PRIVATE JOURNAL
Disability medical exam today.

Brian and I began praying together in earnest for whatever the Lord wants to do about our move to Texas, any ministry opportunities there, selling the house, a place to live there, etc. Brian took authority in Jesus' name and told his left side to wake up.

BRIAN: about the disability exam
I went up to the Disability exam in Winchester March 17, 2017. That was a weird thing. I could tell that although I didn't have anything to try to hide, the man was accustomed to looking for people who were faking. He was very attentive in the way he examined me and watched me walk.

However, as soon as he called me back to his office, I could tell that he discerned, "Oh, okay. This one's for real." He had me do a couple little things, but then he said, "All right. I can see there's no problem here. I'm not the one who makes the final determination; I simply let them know what I see during the examination." I told him what had been going on, whre I was feeling, what I was able to do and not do. He asked me about my career before, where I used to work, etc.

Coming home I struggled with the idea of, "Am I going to 'own' disability? Am I going to say, 'Yes, I am disabled'? Will I accept the label of 'disability'? Or am I going to claim God's provision in this way without accepting the label of being disabled?"

While I was praying about it, I felt the Lord say, "This isn't permanent. It doesn't mean that you're permanently disabled. But for now, right now, take the money. You've earned it; you've worked for it." My therapists were always quick to remind me, "This is why Disability exists! Not so that people can claim they have an anxiety disorder and need a puppy. It's because of people who have worked their whole lives, paid into it. Then something happens which prohibits them from continuing to work in their chosen profession. Take the Disability. If you get back to where you can work, great! If not, then that's what disability income was designed for." It was as if the Lord was saying, "I've put things in place. I'm moving the hands that decide what happens to you. I'm in all of this. You're not going to, by accepting Disability, tie My hands or resign yourself to a life with a handicap. This is part of My plan. Take it."

I don't believe that this disability is permanent.

Sheila: Well, God told you it wasn't.

Brian: If I get back to work, they'll stop the disability income (SSDI). However, it's there to help. What it's done is allowed me time to focus on my healing and recovery with the Lord, both physically and spiritually.

Sheila: Yes. And do you remember the day before you went to that exam? We had seen your original physician from the rehab center. You were beginning to feel like you didn't need to wear the leg brace all the time, didn't need to use the cane most of the time. When we saw the doctor that day, he directed you to definitely use the cane all the time and definitely wear the leg brace all the time. We didn't necessarily agree with that recommendation—and even some of the therapists had varying opinions regarding braces and canes—but we followed the doctor's directive. So you went to the disability appointment suited up in support hose, a foot brace which went into your left shoe and came halfway up your calf, a padded knee brace, and a cane. You looked probably as "disabled" as you could possibly look that morning, and all under doctor definitive directives. I don't think that was by accident! That probably helped the case to gain disability status, but you weren't trying to be deceitful. You were just following doctor's orders from the day before. Remember that? That was kind of funny, but just another sign of the Lord's perfect timing and intervention.

Brian: Yes. In my mind I was saying, "I don't need this stuff. I need to be strong and power through this, just push through, walk it off." The doctor's point was, "No. Without using that cane and that foot brace, you're damaging your knee." Obviously at a later point in time—several months later I believe—I did quit using those devices. It got to a point that I felt they were becoming more of a hindrance than a help.

ONGOING THERAPY
PROCESS ... NEW DEVELOPMENTS

March 19, 2015

Blessings: food stamps kicked back in since Colton has hardly worked in weeks (construction). He is working again which is good too! We have to count his income since he lives with us.

Enjoyed lunch with a dear friend today! She is one of those friends that you can laugh, cry, and be inspired all at the same time. She and her husband had also been through significant challenges with debt in the past. I so appreciated hearing her God stories!

March 20, 2015

Therapist is saying the ataxia is better today...that's the involuntary shaking that happens to the muscles after a stroke.

March 24, 2015 PUBLIC JOURNAL

I've been so cold lately, especially my legs, just can't get warm. Took my blood pressure tonight. It's 87/64! No wonder I'm cold! Good grief. Too bad Brian and I can't share.

March 24, 2015 PRIVATE JOURNAL

Lord, you told me long ago in dreams and through Scripture that our move/future ministry would not make sense to most people including believers. That we would not have many details beforehand, but that in the going Your plan and provision would be revealed. I believe You. I decide to follow You and heed Your voice even when it doesn't make sense. As things draw closer and these truths are played out, please increase my faith. Give me the words to say or not say when describing it to friends and especially family. In Jesus' name, let me not bow to fear in any way—fear of man, fear of future, fear of rejection ... all those old bondage issues. I am free! Thank you, Jesus!

March 25, 2015

Much encouragement and many reasons to be thankful today....

Day started with fellowship, breakfast, worship, and prayer with a special friend. She had interceded diligently for us during our trip to Texas. It was so neat recounting how the Lord worked and cool to hear what she had heard from the Spirit as she prayed, then seeing how that corresponded to what we were experiencing during the trip.

The man came to fix the basement wall today.

New eval with PT (physical therapist) confirmed the gut feelings Brian and I have been thinking about his foot brace as well as knee brace. Seems like a fresh perspective and some different treatment techniques, which I believe will catapult him to a higher level of functioning! Amazing to hear reports of his level of mobility the first day of therapy compared to today! Thank you, Lord! The PT said the fact that he is still getting new muscle function back eight-and-a-half months after the stroke is pretty incredible and indicates that he will regain a lot of function. (I thought, "Of course, because that's what God said at the beginning!")

Tomorrow we will go see the specialist who made the brace and go from there.

Of course we always have a good time at OT! These excellent therapists come up with new challenges for Brian, and I get to watch him work. Lol

And we got indication today that Disability is moving on a positive direction!

Top off the night with a Bible study and inspirational teaching about not wearing our past from Joshua 4–5.

March 25, 2015 PRIVATE JOURNAL

Significant day of—although Brian hates this word—breakthrough! Brian was able to thank God for the stroke because all the Lord has accomplished. Wow. And he said he felt that since we had been able to pray together prayers of belief and power in Jesus' name, we were now seeing these answers. Later that day we also met with a new PT who has insights for a new brace and methods to continue the healing process in Brian's foot/walking.

Brian sensed that God had told him his healing would be completed after Disability $ kicked in. If he would've been healed right away we would not have gotten the "war renumeration" that the enemy was being forced to pay.

Genesis 50:20 AMP, "As for you, you meant evil against me, but God meant it for good in order to bring about this present outcome, that many people would be kept alive [as they are this day]."

Genesis 50:20 NIV: "You intended to harm me, but God used it for good...."

As far as the move to Texas: I realized that although Brian has received detailed clarity and vision about aspects of our ministry there, I have received very little. The Lord has kept me from having expectations because He knows how I am derailed by them! I can easily become disappointed, confused, distracted, and discouraged. So I am working on blind trust and calm assurance of His leading. (Isaiah 42:16) God has confirmed to me over and over that it will be like Abraham setting out, *"Leave and go to a land I will show you."* (Genesis 12 NLT) In the going will come the provision and the clarity. Help me, Jesus! As far as what house to live in when we get there, my Abba Father has shown me so many times how much He loves me and knows my desires even when I haven't told anyone. He knows what I need, what I think I want. And He knows what is best, what will feed my soul. Thank You, Father.

DECISION TO MOVE
TO TEXAS

March 27, 2015 PRIVATE JOURNAL

At this point the Lord truly has confirmed—over and over in a multitude of ways—our call to move to Fort Davis, Texas. We plan to put the house in the market this Spring. It's in His hands as far as timing, obviously. The hardest part for me is interrupting Garret's school, **but** God loves him more than I do and has all of that in perfect timing. By the way, he turns eighteen tomorrow!!

We will soon make the move a public announcement. It is out of the box and basically a missionary call of sorts. I'm not expecting most people (even believers) to understand. Good thing the Lord healed me of the fear of what people think and need for approval … but it is a decision to continue to walk in that freedom from bondage. I am currently doing the Beth Moore <u>Believing God</u> study again. What a blessing that has been. Very different life circumstances but the same powerful God!

Brian gets frustrated with my processing all of this at times! In his mind I should just get over it and do it. He's right, of course. The bottom line is "Did I feel God's call to move to Fort Davis? Have I personally seen and heard the Lord confirm it?" Yes! Then that's it. There is no explanation needed. Besides, we must obey God. Everything else—money, Garrett, my aging mother, his parents' needs—God is well aware of and will cover those needs. His plans are good plans which give us a future and a hope. He is a God of win-win.

I praise you, Lord. Thank You. I do believe! Please help me, enable me to walk strong in You, in what You are leading us into. Enlarge my faith. Embolden my trust in You. I think of the scripture about the disciple putting the hand to the plow and then looking back... Jesus said, "Follow Me. Let the dead bury their own dead."

> *Luke 9:57–62 NIV: As they were walking along the road, a man said to him, "I will follow you wherever you go." Jesus replied, "Foxes have dens and birds have nests, but the Son of Man has no place to lay his head." He said to another man, "Follow me." But he replied, "Lord, first let me go and bury my father." Jesus said to him, "Let the dead bury their own dead, but you go and proclaim the kingdom of God." Still another said, "I will follow you, Lord; but first let me go back and say goodbye to my family." Jesus replied, "No one who puts a hand to the plow and looks back is fit for service in the kingdom of God."*

My dear friend shared her perspective when she was stepping out in faith and telling people about a significant decision in her life. She said she would ask people, "Do you know me? Do you believe that I hear from God? Do you trust who I am in God?" If the answer is yes, then all I can say is that this is what God is saying. And I must obey." That advice was extremely helpful and encouraging to me.

For me as far as with the timing, selling the house, Garrett and everything else... I don't even know what to ask for. I'm asking for Your perfect plan, Lord, because You do know.

This week through the Believing God study, the Lord reminded me of those in my family line who blazed a trail of faith—in fairly wild ways at times and halfway around the globe not just across the country! Grandma and Grandpa Seymour in the mid-1920s to French Equatorial Africa (later called Chad); their son and wife to build a medical/dental practice also in Chad in the 1960's training natives to run it. And later, their grandson and wife to build a seminary in Chad and train the natives as pastors in the 1980's. Thank you, Lord, for a heritage of faith in those godly examples in my own family! Of course my father's parents, although not missionaries, left their home country of Italy to blaze a new life in America in the early 1900s. The story goes that sometime later, after learning discrepancies of faith in their native religion, they jumped out of the box culturally and developed a strong testimony in Jesus Christ.

I have spent a significant amount of time and energy processing and praying through our sense of "the call of God" as well as my thoughts and feelings about missions from my life's observances through my extended family. Frankly, although I have sincerely wanted to be submitted and used by God, I have always been afraid He would send me to Africa or some other third world remote place. (Fort Davis IS remote, but certainly far from third world!) I have shared many of these thoughts, fears and feelings with my eighty-two-year-old mother. She has been extremely supportive, an encourager and prayer warrior through all this.

March 27, 2015 Brian: THEN reflections

This was after we decided, through our trip February 2015, that—since we still were being called to move to Fort Davis, Texas—we wanted to surrender to God. We had to sit down together and just decide, "Are we still going to do this?" I prayed a lot before I committed to that decision because, you know, an awful lot had happened in our lives since 2012 when we first got an inkling of a call to move West!

First of all, as a man, I was asking the Lord, "How can I do this? I can't move. I can't physically pack the truck and unpack it. I can't do all the things required to move across country. We've lived here for nineteen years. We have a lot of junk! I have a three--bay garage." That was one huge issue on my mind. Another was, "How are we going to make a living? What are we going to live on? Disability was coming through, but it wasn't that much every month."

Sheila: And at this point we still had the debt payments. They hadn't been taken care of yet.

Brian: And where are we going to live? How will we afford rent or to buy a house? How are things going to work out financially? How are we going to survive? And then...plus Garrett! What's Garrett going to do there? We're going to a town much smaller even than Edinburg, VA. What will there be for Garrett?" All these things were pressing on my mind. So I offered up a couple fleeces to God. I never told anybody what they were, not even Sheila. I never said them out loud. It was just between me and God because I thought I heard God say, "Here's where I'm calling you, Brian, if you're willing to take this step. I know this is a **huge** step for you, way outside the box. I know I'm asking you to make a big step. If you can't do it, I'll understand. I'll still use you where you are. It's not as though you'll be in punishment or that I'll put you in the corner until you obey. It's not like that. Rather, here is an opportunity—if you want to see a bigger Me, then follow. If you want to get a bigger perspective on Me, take this step. I'll understand if you can't because I'm asking you to take a big step of faith. But I'm giving you a chance to do this."

I remember telling Sheila that, and we prayed about it. We both agreed that we were willing to try it. Why not? What's the worst that can happen—we have to come back with our tail between our legs and say that we hadn't heard from God or made a mistake? No. We didn't believe that would be the case at all, so we decided to try it. I didn't know exactly the timeframe because we knew there were some things we'd have to prepare before making a big move like that—house projects, for example. At that point, Sheila and I decided that we were probably going to put the house on the market in the Spring and follow this journey the Lord was laying out.

*** *I vividly remember the decision making process of moving across the country. Sure, there was an aspect of being weary of the stroke trauma and the recovery process ... wanting to go somewhere **new** and get a fresh start. However, we held each other accountable and prayed countless times for the Lord to **not** let that be our main motivation! We only wanted to make this huge move if it truly was His hand leading us.*

Just a couple days ago I was talking to a dear friend I met out here (in Alpine, Texas, but she actually grew up not far from my hometown in Pennsylvania—small world) about how once you make the decision to stretch your wings at God's prompting and take a leap of faith a couple thousand miles across the country, it becomes easier to make the leap once again—to wherever God may lead. Why not? It's a big world, the Lord owns it all, and many adventures await! We have experienced a sense of freedom I don't believe would have come otherwise.

Trusting The Lord Through The Financial Issues

March 30, 2015

In the midst of a jam-packed day today, I found myself praying (**again**) to surrender to the Lord's plans, not to get so wound tight that I think it's up to me to control or plan or organize the next steps. My shoulders and neck are super tight, which are reminders to me to **stop**, surrender, pray for peace, and **rest** in Jesus. Thankful that His mercies are new every morning!

March 31, 2015 PRIVATE JOURNAL

Brian asked me to pray this morning. In so doing, the Holy Spirit gave me this: the walk that he is struggling with is both physical and spiritual. God is teaching him a new way to walk. That resonated deeply with Brian.

We got word today verifying the amount of money coming with Disability. It wasn't as much in the lump sum as we thought, but it's OK! God knows what we need! It was such a blessing to have the answer come forth. And yet what was interesting to me was that it did not really feel like a "weight lifted" but rather just another step, another revelation, another example of God's provision.

*** *And looking back, honestly that's how it felt: just another step, another part of the journey. From the beginning of the stroke experience it seemed so obvious to me that we were on a journey. Were there times I was discouraged or frustrated or deeply sad or concerned? Absolutely! However, it was incredibly evident to me that the Lord was holding us very closely and directing each step of the way. That is part of the reason I journaled so avidly throughout—I sensed we would want to be able to look back on this process in detail, tracing how God worked in us and through us. I also had the feeling early on that the story would become more public and in book form to share on a broad scale. For me to have the idea of writing a book is not surprising. When Brian stated he thought we were supposed to write a book, I knew that was God!*

March 31, 2015 PUBLIC JOURNAL
Check out 2 Corinthians 1:9–11...thank you to those of you who have kept praying for us, and thanks be to God who never fails!!

2 Corinthians 1:8–11 NIV: "We do not want you to be uninformed, brothers and sisters, about the troubles we experienced in the province of Asia. We were under great pressure, far beyond our ability to endure, so that we despaired of life itself. Indeed, we felt we had received the sentence of death. But this happened that we might not rely on ourselves but on God, who raises the dead. He has delivered us from such a deadly peril, and he will deliver us again. On him we have set our hope that he will continue to deliver us, as you help us by your prayers. Then many will give thanks on our behalf for the gracious favor granted us in answer to the prayers of many."

The timing of the Lord never ceases to amaze me. What might seem delayed in our minds is not a delay to His Sovereign plan.

Last Wednesday we got a call from Social Security stating that Brian had been approved for Disability! **Yes**! We were so thankful for this relatively quick answer (quick in the world of government—only eight months). The message said we needed to call back to provide some additional information regarding a minor child on the account (Garrett). Since that day we have called numerous times, left voicemail messages to no avail. Yesterday morning when we tried, there was an automated message saying the office was closed. We were in Winchester yesterday so we drove by the office. Yep. Closed. Government holiday? Not that we could figure out. This morning the same closed message was on the automated voicemail. So ... we called the Harrisonburg SS office. Guess what? Yes, the Winchester SS office will be closed for thirty days because mold was discovered in the building. The phones were supposed to relay that information and forward the calls to the Harrisonburg office. That did not happen. **But** Brian got to speak with a very kind woman this morning, lay out our situation **and** get answers. Thank you, Lord!

A lump sum is on its way to our bank account. That is payment for January, February, and March. Then we will receive monthly payment hereafter. We had thought we would receive back pay from the date we applied for disability (7/27/14), but that is not the case. You have to be disabled for five months before the payments kick in. **It's OK**. God knows the amount we need, and we are **praising** Him for the provision!

Things were getting rather tight, money drained from other accounts. Even so, we have always had what we need. God promises that.

I'd like to share one neat experience: back in July or August we received a large love gift from a church. I cashed the check into $50s and would just take one out periodically as needed or as the Lord directed. I never did count the remaining money in that envelop; I felt that I was not supposed to count it but just trust that God would make it last as long as necessary. I've had to dip into it more often lately. However, there are still $50 bills in that envelop! It reminds me of the woman in the Old Testament with the jar of oil that didn't run out. She continued doing what God directed her to do using the oil to serve the prophet and her family as needed. God made the oil stretch and last until other provision was made available. (1 Kings 17 and 2 Kings 4)

At times it was tempting to want to count the money in the envelop, in order to humanly discern how much was available. But so much more thrilling it has been to watch how God provides!

For anyone who knows my past struggle with being in control, having a plan and my own expectations—this is a testimony to healing and deliverance! Go Jesus!

Continuing In
"The Process"

April 3, 2015

I noticed the scripture today: Exodus 24:1 NIV, *"Come up to the Lord ... [but] worship at a distance."* This is very different from what we see in Revelation 4:1 NIV, *"Come up here."* Because of Jesus we have full access to the presence of the Father! Because of Jesus, the One who saves. Hosanna! Which means, "Save us. Save now."

April 4, 2015

Brian wants to issue a special thank-you to our local family doctor, for "making my wife impossible to live with! Our doctor told her she was amazing! As if she needed confirmation, she now has a doctor's note! This statement was made because she had not only lost weight since her last checkup but her lab work was excellent. Doctor said she has the blood pressure of a teenager! Good grief. Maybe we can exchange some!"

April 4, 2015. Recorded while he was putting together a model car:

BRIAN:

Hello. Sheila's doing a video of me doing my miniature cars. I just finished up a '57 Ford two-door sedan. I don't know. Just something to pass the time and keep my hand working. It's something kind of fun. I can have a lot of cars this way!

Sheila: Oh, brother!

Brian: It doesn't cost me much. I think that one turned out pretty good, not "Amazing" like Sheila's doctor report! God is good and things are moving along pretty well. I don't know what to tell you except that He's faithful and true. Everything that you read about Him in the Bible is true. I don't know what else I can tell you except encourage you to read it for yourself. Find out what it says. Because it really makes a difference. He promises to always take care of us. Always look out for us and never leave us—even in the midst of struggles. Especially in the midst of struggles.

April 6, 2015

I spent time today reflecting on how, over the years, the Lord has been moving Brian and me out of the box in regards to church, ministry, and life. Even going back to how we met and our dating relationship as teenagers, our decisions about careers—which were unconventional—shaped our growth as dreamers, entrepreneurs, and people who desperately wanted to avoid the rut of life.

In 1996 God brought us to the Shenandoah Valley in Virginia. We continued to grow here and expand in ministry. There have been so many events during these years, not to mention the birth of Garrett and our entrance into the world of parenting special needs children. We have seen the good, the bad, the ugly, as well as the marvelous in aspects of ministry and Christian community. Through it all the Lord has continued to shape and mold us, faithfully opening our eyes more and more to the gifts of the Spirit and the uniquely mysterious moves of God. Particularly significant during this time were the years we spent most every weekend at the Christian coffee shop in Edinburg, fellowshipping with people from all over the country, all different churches and walks of life, and learning to worship with musicians from all genres.

This confirmed a sense we'd had for years that God was calling us to a ministry to the Church in general, not to one local congregation long term. The connections that were made during that time cannot be over-stated! Then in 2012 God laid "Guerrilla Worship" on Brian's heart, and we embarked on a whole new spiritual frontier. In Guerrilla Worship we would drive around prayerfully until we sensed a place God wanted us to stop. Brian, guitar in hand, would walk the area and pray as led by the Holy Spirit over the land, the community or however God led. We had some fascinating experiences!

We spent some brief but rich time at a small church in Woodstock, Virginia, soaking in worship music led by others, the Word, and people who believed Jesus and walked it out, instead of just talking about it on Sundays. It was a season of healing and restoration in our lives. (As worship leaders for years, we had been through extreme spiritual warfare including wounding at the hands of other Christians in the church. As a result, we were burned-out, bruised, disillusioned with traditional church, and weary in soul and spirit. Although those experiences were incredibly painful, we are thankful for them because we can relate to so many indi-viduals who get wounded in the very place they go seeking healing, the church.) *** *If this hits home to you, we would love to minister to you personally. Please contact us at sheilalloydlive2@yahoo.com*

Also in 2012 we met missionary Paula Evans from Fort Davis, Texas. The Lord had led her for a season to Edinburg, Virginia. The friendship with Paula was one of those amazing connections God brought to us through a little Christian coffee shop. Through her ministry of prayer counseling and God-given insights, the Lord did major healing work in my life—in ways too deep to explain in this context. The Lord used her unconventional but sold-out faith to draw us closer to His heart. It was a time in our spiritual lives, as I alluded to above, where we were seeking something deeper than anything we had experienced in traditional church settings. We also heard of how God was moving in the Big Bend area as well as Sunspot, NM, and our hearts were absolutely set ablaze. So after much prayer, we decided to visit in August 2013, and we felt the call of God.

We realized that we were considering a radical change of lifestyle. Brian phrased it like this on the trip home in August 2013: "I believe the Lord is saying, 'Hey guys, I'm getting ready to do some really cool stuff out here. I would love to have you be a part of it if you can make the leap. It's your choice, though. If you feel it's too big of a change, I will still love you where you are. I will bless you and continue to use you in ministry where you are. But if you want to take a leap, it would be a lot of fun to have you join me.'" Truly we felt we had a choice. (Now certainly there are times that the Lord commands and you simply answer, "Yes, Sir!" He is God Almighty after all. This instance was a different situation.) But we had both determined long before that if the Lord asked anything of us, our answer would be, "Yes, Lord!" Brian's imagery in this prayer was of stepping off a cliff believing the Lord was the only safety net.

The stroke came July 10, 2014 after we have decided to put our house on the market and move to Texas. What has followed is simply more of the journey … Full surrender of our dreams, our future, our expectations … and giving control to Jesus Christ our Lord. God was/is doing a radically new thing in every area of our lives!

Isaiah 43:18–19 NIV: *"Forget the former things; do not dwell on the past. See, I am doing a new thing! Now it springs up; do you not perceive it? I am making a way in the wilderness and streams in the wasteland."*

Father, I confess at times I still rebel against it. Not my will but Yours be done. Please help me.

April 8, 2015
Check out Romans chapters 7 and 8 in *The Message* version. Wow! New perspective.

NINTH MONTH MARK

April 10, 2015
Well, it's been nine months today since Brian had the stroke.

*** *I'll admit it was sobering every month when we hit that mark. I would often feel a little sad and frankly, a little surprised that God hadn't yet brought the full healing. Oh, I understood that it was a process and that we were on a journey. And certainly we were seeing His hand all over the circumstances, but I just wanted to jump to the end of the journey—let's get to the victory part, the part where Brian is miraculously and completely healed! Now after three-plus years, I realize the journey is the victory. The process is the miracle—watching, feeling, living the lessons the Lord has taught/is teaching in us, and how He has used/is using our story to minister to others. I still believe God will completely heal and restore Brian, but I have a slightly different perspective on what full healing and restoration mean. Physical healing is only one layer.*

The last couple weeks have been very interesting—Brian had significant revelations from the Lord leading to resolutions within himself just in the 24 hours before we heard that Disability had been approved. God's timing never ceases to amaze me.

Even before we received the positive Disability decision, we both sensed that we had rounded a corner in this process … maybe it had to do with going on our trip to Texas, maybe it had to do with winter breaking and seeing signs of Spring, maybe both of those with a myriad of other spiritual influences... but it was a welcomed realization for both of us.

A couple weeks ago we earnestly prayed together that the Lord would give wisdom about how to proceed with his foot. He felt like he had reached a plateau of sorts. That prayer was answered, and we have been working that new approach. Brian feels that the Lord shows him step by step what to focus on. For example, last week he realized that if he works **really** hard stretching out his left shoulder almost to the point of exhaustion, then he has a lot more fine motor control in his left hand for playing guitar. I admire him for continuing to exercise every day and persevere in his therapy. We hear encouragement from therapists such as, "I have to constantly devise new things for you each time you come in because you keep achieving the goals I set for you" and "The fact that you are getting new movement and new sensation this long after the stroke is a rather unusual but wonderful sign that you will regain lots of strength." (I know. Full recovery. That's what God said.)

No doubt about it, our world was turned upside down July 10 when he had that stroke. It has been an interesting, albeit quite difficult, journey adjusting to new realities. Despite the tough times, there have truly been many, many blessings and enriching lessons in the midst of it all!

Often in the moments when I would feel overwhelmed that, "Holy crap! My forty-six-year-old husband had a stroke!" I would be reminded that many other people go through injuries, sicknesses, etc., which require long-term healing and perseverance on the journey. There are tons of physical therapists, occupational therapists, orthotics specialists—just to name a few fields—whose full time careers serve individuals who are on a long-term recovery program! My mother had a minor fall December 28 which progressed into a severe wound, her leg in danger, cellulitis, therapy, and being basically shut in her home for about three months! She is still making weekly trips to the wound clinic. (A whole clinic devoted to wounds!) I guess my point is that although, yes, a stroke is drastic, people face many challenges in life which require a **process** of healing.

Isn't the same thing true for our spiritual lives? Our emotional well-being? We must go through a process of realization, choosing to change and then an intentional pursuit of growth. For those who choose Jesus Christ as Lord and Savior, **He** does the work in us. We must choose to surrender to the process, to His loving hand and sanctification. We go through transformation.

2 Corinthians 3:12–18 NIV: *"Therefore, since we have such a hope, we are very bold. We are not like Moses, who would put a veil over his face to prevent the Israelites from seeing the end of what was passing away. But their minds were made dull, for to this day the same veil remains when the old covenant is read. It has not been removed, because only in Christ is it taken away. Even to this day when Moses is read, a veil covers their hearts. But whenever anyone turns to the Lord, the veil is taken away. Now the Lord is the Spirit, and where the Spirit of the Lord is, there is freedom. And we all, who with unveiled faces contemplate the Lord's glory, are being transformed into his image with ever-increasing glory, which comes from the Lord, who is the Spirit."*

BRIAN: God wanted to get me alone with Him.

You were saying that Jesus does the work. As I was coming on a year out from the stroke, I started to see all the things that God has done in our lives (a) to help in my recovery—the things He's allowing me to get back, and (b) activities He's giving me the time to do. I've had time to study the Bible, to spend with Him that I never thought I had the time to do before. It's almost as if He had to get me alone with Him. He wanted my undivided attention, and I wasn't listening before.

Not that I'm saying He caused the stroke as a punishment. God knew the stroke was coming because He's God. He knows everything that happens. Also, the enemy knew that we had decided after our trip in 2013 that we were going to move to Fort Davis, Texas. We made no secret about that. We had flown out to visit a missionary friend and investigate the other ways we'd heard the Lord was moving in the area. After we got home and through more prayer, we had made up our minds that we were going to move. It's almost as though Satan did not want that to happen, so—kind of like Job— he wanted to test us. (The devil cannot read our minds, but he certainly is astute to our words and actions. We make our intentions very clear. We also make our fears and weaknesses very clear…something to consider. Also, see Job chapters 1–2, Satan has to get permission from the Father before beginning those horrible trials in Job's life.)

Satan wanted to test our faith, to see how well we would really cling to God. So the enemy gave me the stroke; I think Satan caused it. And God, like with Job, said, "Okay, you can do this, Satan, but you can't take his mind; and you can't take his life." I fully believe that.

Sheila: I totally believe that. Well, you were even talking about Job as the stroke was happening! You were saying, "Just like Job had to learn that God was number one … nothing else mattered. Not his wife or his children or his livelihood. Nothing was of higher importance than God in his life. And I feel that way. Satan can throw whatever he wants at me. I will not deny Jesus Christ. Jesus is number one in my life!" You had tears in your eyes while you were saying it, which I chalked up to the Holy Spirit laying that on your heart so strongly. Later, a friend who was there said the added emotion could have also been part of the beginning of the stroke. A moment after those words came out of your mouth, I noticed your having trouble chewing the snack.

Brian: One thing I was learning more and more at this time (almost a year after the stroke) was this idea of surrender—relinquishing your life and your dreams to God. God knows who I am and what I personally like, what I enjoy doing. But He also knows who He wants me to be. When you surrender, instead of clinging on to what you think is your identity—"God, You made me this way. I'm a _____. I have to do _____." That attitude doesn't allow God to shape you. God was shaping me into something different. I still look the same and talk the same, and I'm still interested in the same things. However, I have a much different perspective on those things as God is moving me and showing me how to truly let go.

Part of that is, as events took place, I started seeing the hand of God. You start sitting there, watching it happen, saying, "My God. I couldn't have made that happen! I couldn't have brought about that outcome—for example with phone calls to creditors or financial aid for hundreds of thousands of dollars owed to hospitals—and You just did it! You made it happen in the perfect time. I wanted it six months ago, but You knew that actually now we'd be at the point where it needed to happen. It's the perfect time." So you learn to just take your hands off and let God drive because knows where He's going. I don't. I don't know where God's going. I just know when God says, "Hey, do this," I do it.

You don't ask questions. You don't say, "Why, God?" Now, you can ask why later, "Why did You have me do that, Lord?" But many times it will have become clear because you see how things worked out. You realize, "Oh, that's why." Beforehand you don't know. That's part of trust. That's part of faith. I know that my Father loves me. I'm reminded of a plaque a friend gave me while I was in rehab—"God will not take you where His grace cannot keep you." He's not going to lead you to a place where His grace will not protect you. He won't take you there if He's not going to protect you! Because He is our Protector. He is Protection. He is Provision. He **is** all those things. Even when you pray and want to rebuke the devil in Jesus' name. No. Say to the enemy, "Jesus is rebuking you." I'm not doing it. I'm not rebuking you in Jesus' name. Jesus is doing it, Satan. He's just using me to do it.

Sheila: But Jesus tells us to cast out demons.

Brian: Yes, but if I say, "I cast you out in Jesus' name," that means I'm doing it. It's something He's showing me—another way to give Him glory. Not drawing the attention to myself. I need to have the authority—given to me by Christ—to say, "Jesus Christ casts you out." It's all Christ.

Brian is not the same man he was nine months ago. I am not the same woman. Our marriage is not the same. By the grace of God we are stronger, more surrendered, more in love, and more devoted to Jesus and to one another. Thank you, Lord.

Hmmmmm … nine months. The time of a normal pregnancy. Wonder what God is birthing. Sounds like I have my next topic of Bible study.

BIBLE STUDY AND SPIRITUAL INSIGHTS

April 13, 2015 PRIVATE JOURNAL

A huge part of this process for me has been recognizing God is wanting to develop a servant's heart in me. A heart of humility, of compassion, and a life embodied by service are truly representative of Jesus. This has not been an easy surgery for me.

Revelation: When I was whining internally about my plans being thwarted again to meet someone else's agenda (even though that someone was my husband), the old song came to mind, "Broken and Spilled Out." Jesus, who do you want to be to me today, in this moment? He reminded me that He was constantly setting aside His own needs for the sake of those He loved! Following a higher agenda, He pursued the salvation of our souls. How many times, Jesus, did You serve in sheer exhaustion and even frustration? Were there times You didn't have the "want to," the energy reserves?

In the last several years we have had prophecies, words of encouragement, and I have had several dreams about being "pregnant"—that God was birthing something in us or through us. I did some interesting study in Scripture in relation to that concept. This was at the nine-month mark: it has been nine months since the stroke. So I have wondered what the Lord has been preparing us for, what this "pregnancy" over the last few years is leading up to.

Here are some of my conclusions from that study: In my own strength I can "birth" nothing of any value. It's only wind; it does not bring salvation. What is brought forth in our own strength is easily destroyed by ourselves! And so I prayed, "Dear Lord, fill me with your strength to give birth to whatever you have destined for me." John 3:6 NIV says, "*Flesh gives birth to flesh, but the Spirit gives birth to spirit.*" In other words it's His plan not mine.

And so I asked the Holy Spirit, "What are some things that the Lord was pregnant with for a season? Things that took time to set into action? Or that there was a process before something was birthed?" (If this is a foreign concept to you—about asking the Holy Spirit, does the Bible not say that he dwells inside us and that his number one goal is to guide us into all truth? See John 16:12–15; 14:17. And the Bible clearly says if anyone lacks wisdom he should ask God who gives freely to all without finding fault. See James 1:5. I have found that the Holy Spirit gives me amazing insights when I take the time to ask Him, and then wait on Him to reveal.)

Here are some things that the Lord was pregnant with for a season. These events took time to set into action; there was a process before something was birthed.

* The plan of redemption through Jesus Christ! God waited roughly 4,000 years from the Garden of Eden. And yet amidst the curses implemented in Genesis 3, a Messiah was prophesied.
* Noah built the ark ... more than 100 years before the flood came
* How many years and processes did Joseph go through before God raised him up, and he in turn rescued Israel? This was the bloodline the Messiah would come from.
* The upbringing and positioning of Moses, Esther, Samuel, Daniel to name a few! How often did it involve trials? Every time.

* Joshua was mentored by Moses to become a leader, as was Elisha with Elijah.
* There was a long period of time between when David was anointed as a young man and when he took over the role as king over united Israel and Judah. God was birthing a king who would have character—a warrior, a psalter, a worshiper, one who would lead by example, not a perfect man but one after God's own heart. It took time for the Lord to prepare one who would establish a righteous kingdom and also methods of worship in the tabernacle of holy design.
* Jonah—the time between his calling, rebellion, and transformation to humility and his acceptance of God's way, which allowed him to see a mighty move of God.
* Elizabeth, who as an old woman became pregnant with John the Baptist. Her pregnancy overlapped Mary's. Elizabeth was in preparation to parent the one Jesus said was greater than any man who ever lived. And John the Baptist prepared the way for the Messiah.
* And the disciples spent three years with Jesus in preparation to "birth" the spread of the Gospel into all the world!

*** *Even today, two-and-a-half years after this writing, it is so encouraging to read this!*

April 13, 2015 PUBLIC JOURNAL

My God is able to do abundantly more than I can ask or even imagine!

Ephesians 3:20–21 NIV: *"Now to him who is able to do immeasurably more than all we ask or imagine, according to his power that is at work within us, to him be glory in the church and in Christ Jesus throughout all generations, for ever and ever! Amen."*

April 16, 2015

> Matthew 11:28–30 NIV: *"Come to me, all you who are weary and burdened, and I will give you rest. Take my yoke upon you and learn from me, for I am gentle and humble in heart, and you will find rest for your souls. For my yoke is easy and my burden is light."*

April 17, 2015

There is so much **more** going on over our heads than we realize ... applies certainly in the spiritual realm but often played out on the physical realm if we have eyes to see and ears to hear.

April 18, 2015

At a point in time when I was desperate for some refreshment and quiet time, the Lord provided a way that I could attend a women's retreat. It was held at the beautiful Young Life campus in Rockbridge, Virginia, nestled in the mountains. I took copious notes partly because it helps my rather active mind stay focused, partly because the Holy Spirit was speaking volumes to me and I wanted to capture it. Full permission was granted from the speaker, Claire Hetrick, for me to include these notes.

The speaker shared of a close friend of hers struggling with a terminal illness. Sitting by her friend's bedside at one point, she heard her weakened voice say in a whisper, "Why me, Lord?" Shocked because her friend had not complained at all about her illness, she leaned closer. The sick woman said once again, "Why me, Lord?" And then said, "This is so beautiful! Why me, Lord?"

The speaker, Claire Hetrick, proceeded to tie this in with the story of Lazarus' death in John chapter 11. Jesus received the news that Lazarus was dying, but he waited two more days before he traveled there. Jesus loved them so much, and therefore He waited two more days. Jesus comes when the time is right. But the sisters say, "If you had been here...." Jesus knew he was going to raise Lazarus from the dead, but the sisters didn't. They still had to go all through the pain of the death. Lazarus had to go through final breath. What was the purpose? The glory of God! Jesus goes into Bethany knowing it would mean his death, but that was all part of God's plan. Jesus is going toward his crucifixion … and his resurrection. Lazarus' resurrection was a foreshadowing of our resurrection in Christ. The sisters didn't see any point in Jesus waiting two days. If Jesus had come right away, their brother would not have died. True, but the greater purpose of the lesson of faith would not have been learned by the sisters, by Lazarus, or by us. This talk ministered to me greatly at this time—waiting for the Lord to heal Brian.

Here are some other notes from that talk:

Jesus meets three people outside Bethany, and they all question his motives. To Mary, Jesus gives truth. To Martha, Jesus gives hope. And to the mourners, Jesus displays action and power. Jesus says, "I am what you need"—that is, the glory of God. So the question is, "Do you believe?" Martha says yes even before Lazarus is raised. Does Jesus see that faith in me? The miracles show the glory of God. And it's not that **God** needs the glory. I need the glory. Jesus shows himself to me when life is the darkest, in my pain. Jesus was moved by Martha's pain. He weeps for Israel. Jesus weeps for Israel in pain, and he weeps for me. I believe he still weeps for all of us because we haven't quite understood yet. Do I sense Jesus' compassion for me?

Later in her talk, Claire posed another question, "What needs to be buried that will allow Jesus' resurrection in my life?" And she brought up Romans 8:28 NIV, *"All things work together for good to those who love God and are called according to his purpose."* But then she made a statement which I found true although we don't think of it this way enough. Claire said, "We need to define good the way God defines good." That really resonated with me in regards to our current situation! Then she asked, "Do you really know the Lord? Because you will never trust the stranger, even if that stranger is God. So if I'm having trouble finding God's mercy in the situation, then go back and get to know the Shepherd more."

There were many statements that weekend that the Holy Spirit used to minister to my heart. And I'm not trying to steal somebody else's insights, but I'm just trying to give you a picture of where I was emotionally and spiritually.

Besides the obvious things on my mind involving Brian's recovery, I was also listening and receiving confirmations about God's moving us to Fort Davis, Texas. One such statement was the following: "God's Kingdom is actually a small kingdom. Geography and time mean nothing in God's kingdom. His Kingdom is everywhere and crosses all boundaries." That was very helpful to a girl who's always been close to her family looking at moving 1,800 miles away.

April 20, 2015

My forty-seventh birthday. A wonderful present:

Results from Brian's OT eval today show current status compared to October 8 eval. Great improvements! Glory to God! Thanks to our wonderful therapists!

April 22, 2015 Facebook post as I was re-reading my notes and still soaking in the nuggets from the retreat:

I was blessed this past weekend to attend a women's retreat. Here are some of my notes:

4/18/2015 Claire Hetrick, speaker at Women's Weekend Rockbridge Alum Springs Young Life Camp

TRUTH – only God's word is truth! And in it we find everything about life and godliness.

She's been studying the miracles of Jesus lately. If you need a miracle in your life, don't pursue the miracle. Pursue the One who does the miracle! Pursue Jesus.

Purpose of the miracles according to Jesus' own words: that you may believe and have life (John 20:30). Jesus said the work of God is to believe in the One He sent (John 6)

Claire said she is a questioner by nature, and so often employs that method when studying the Scripture too. And often the Lord asks her questions! (I have put those questions in CAPS)

If miracles display the glory of God…*DOES MY LIFE REFLECT THAT I BELIEVE?*

The response of people after this miracle was that they believed who Jesus was and thus he began his ministry. *WHAT IS MY RESPONSE TO JESUS FOR WHAT HE HAS DONE IN MY LIFE?*

WHAT DO I KNOW OF GOD? I must hold on to those things in the midst of hard times! She gave an example of a father who took his young child along on a fun weekend of riding four wheelers. By a freak accident, the child was killed. When that man had to call home to tell his wife, he said, "Honey, I need to tell you something really terrible, but before I do, I want you to fill your mind with everything you know about the goodness of God." We live in a fallen world. Bad things do happen to good people, to godly people. We must *KNOW* Jesus and have the goodness of God as the screen through which we face the hard times. (Obviously, this hit home to me!) The raising of Lazarus in John 11 is the last recorded miracle before Jesus' crucifixion and resurrection in Jerusalem. It is the seventh miracle listed in John, and we know that seven is God's number of completion or perfection. So we can say that this miracle is a prologue of what the Lord wants to do in MY life.

WHAT DOES THIS MIRACLE SHOW?

- Shows Jesus' power over death—and therefore, my hope for Heaven. *WHAT DOES MY HOPE LIE IN?*
- Defines the love of the Father – shows how much Jesus loves this family (vs 5). *DO I REFER TO MYSELF AS THE ONE JESUS LOVES?* The Bible states multiple times how much Jesus loved this family (Martha, her sister Mary, and their brother Lazarus), and yet we really do not know too much about them. There are just brief incidents recorded in scripture about them. *HOW MUCH DO I NOT KNOW ABOUT JESUS?*

- People Jesus love *DO* experience suffering. Bad things point to the glory of God. Jesus had a higher purpose than them being in pain. *HOW MUCH AM I WILLING TO SUFFER SO THAT SOMEONE CAN COME TO JESUS?*

At this point, Claire (the speaker), shared a personal story about her dear friend Mary, who fought a very difficult five-year battle with breast cancer and who had died recently. Claire said she had the privilege of walking much of that journey with her, including her last moments here on this earth. Mary had a form of breast cancer in which she had open sores all over the chest that would bleed all the time, so she would hold a towel across her chest. Claire said one day towards the end Mary was not talking much, but Claire saw her mouth moving. Mary was clutching the bloody towel to her chest. Claire leaned in close to hear what she was saying, and heard her say, "Why me, Lord?" Wrecked with emotion, Claire agonized in her spirit. It was the first time in the five-year journey that she had heard Mary ask this question. Claire cried out in her heart to the Lord, "Please give me something to say to comfort her!" However, she heard nothing from Him to say; and as she said, "Thankfully I didn't insert anything of my own." A few moments later she heard Mary say, "This is so beautiful, Lord! Why me?" *WOW*. Claire said, "My friend, you must being seeing something very different than what I'm seeing right now." Indeed, Mary was seeing the *GLORY* of God.

We are told that Jesus loved Lazarus' family so much. The Bible says he received word, "The one you love is sick," and yet he stayed where he was two more days. *WHY DID JESUS WAIT?* One reason: study reveals the Jewish belief at the time was that when a person died, the soul remained with the body for four days. Jesus did not raise Lazarus until he had been dead four days. There could be no doubt—he was "dead dead." *WHY DID JESUS WAIT?* Jesus comes when the time is right. He tells his disciples in John 11:14–15 that it is good that he is not there so they may *BELIEVE*. The sisters go out to meet him outside the town, and this question is the first thing on their lips, "If you had been here, he wouldn't have died." Jesus knew that he was going to raise Lazarus from the dead, thus giving glory to God and fostering belief in those around. *BUT* the sisters didn't know this. Lazarus didn't know this. They still had to go through the pain of death. *WHAT WAS THE PURPOSE?* The Glory of God!

(This particular section really ministered to me. From the first hours of Brian's stroke, I believed that the Lord had spoken to my spirit saying, "He will be completely restored." It has seemed like a very long process of recovery, even though we know in truth it has been miraculously speedy. But still the waiting for "full healing, full restoration" gets difficult at times. Through this story of Lazarus and of Mary saying, "Why me, Lord" seeing the glory of God, the Holy Spirit brought encouragement to my heart and renewed my spirit. Indeed Brian and I have witnessed the glory of God in countless ways these last nine-plus months!)

Jesus says *I AM* what you need! *THAT* is the Glory of God. Jesus asks, *DO YOU BELIEVE?* Martha says yes even before Lazarus is raised. Jesus saw in her a true disciple of faith. *WHAT DOES JESUS SEE IN ME?*

Miracles show the glory of God—it's *NOT* that God needs the glory. I need the glory!

Jesus shows himself to me when life is the darkest, in my pain. Jesus was moved by Martha's pain. He weeps (John 11:35). He knew he was going to raise Lazarus from the dead, so *WHY DID JESUS WEEP?* He wept for their pain; he wept for Israel; he wept because he knew they just hadn't quite "gotten it" yet. He weeps for me. *DO I SEE JESUS' COMPASSION FOR ME?*

Life is about pointing people to Jesus! *WHO DOES MY LIFE POINT TO? DOES MY LIFE POINT PEOPLE TO GOD?*

Jesus raised Lazarus from the dead *JUST LIKE* he will raise me *IF* I believe. This last miracle foreshadows Jesus' resurrection and the culmination of His plan.

As he called to Lazarus, Jesus calls to me, "Sheila, come out of the tomb!" He calls to each of us. Insert your own name. Remove the grave clothes. Jesus offers a second chance, new life! (2 Cor. 5:17) Rejoice! *CAN I HEAR HIM CALLING?*

Remind myself of the resurrection every day. We are called from death to *ABUNDANT* life! (John 10:10)

WHAT NEEDS TO BE BURIED THAT WILL ALLOW JESUS TO BE RESURRECTED IN MY LIFE?

DO I BELIEVE? Jesus gives my joy back, my smile back, my life back from the grave! He says, "You are precious and treasured in my sight, and I love you."

April 22, 2015 PRIVATE JOURNAL:
Arriving home from that weekend, I shared many of Claire Hetrick's insights with Brian. He appreciated them as well. And he made the following comments:

"I had surrendered to the process very early on in the stroke. God is taking this opportunity to bless. He alone is the Sole Provider. He alone is enough. Not the government, not the SSDI (disability income), not people's generosity. Very few people get to see Him to this extent because most people do not let go. God had the grace enough to make me let go. I am the most free I have ever felt because I don't have anyone pulling my strings. He's showing me right now how to live free. He knew I would need this process (the stroke) to learn that lesson. Yes, I believe I will eventually do something, work in some way again. The Bible clearly values work. But I have learned that I don't depend on my own provision."

April 23, 2015
Brian says this morning, "I truly can do all things for it's Christ who strengthens me!" (Phil 4:13 NIV)

April 24, 2015

Brian felt he was ready to get rid of the ramp by the studio and just have a stoop. So thank you, Jerry Wilson and Colton! And when the sunshine returns, Colton will be taking down the ramp into the house. We are **so** grateful to the Lord for continued progress and healing! **Please pray** specifically for full range of motion and control in his left ankle/hip, as well of course as his left hand for the guitar. God is so good. We continue to be humbled by how many people are still thinking of us and praying.

April 25, 2015

Going to miss Challenger baseball this morning. Garrett and I are struggling with allergies, plus it's the first morning in ages that we don't have any agenda.

So I slept in and then have been in living room helping Brian with some new exercises from his PT. They are some ways of stretching out his ankle, leg and hip muscles that I have to help him with. We have worship songs playing on YouTube.

April 27, 2015

Brian has a recheck from his sinus surgery today at UVA....Check this out: the **snot** survey! Too funny!

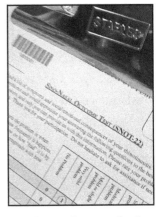

Got him a new I AM SECOND bracelet ... the other one was worn out!

*** *There have been many times on this journey that people have looked at me and said comments like these: "How are you doing this really? How do you do it?" Or this: "Obviously your faith is very strong. I wish mine was as strong as yours, but it's not." (As though I have exclusive rights to the faith market!) Here's a journal entry that was written yesterday, although it could be inserted in many, many places within this book as well!*

October 19, 2017
There are days—like today actually—when I just feel like it's been too much. I'm tired physically and emotionally, very weary of the roller coaster. At the time of this writing, just within the last few weeks, there's been such a swing of events and emotions: family vacation drive across country, fiftieth wedding anniversary celebration, wonderful times reconnecting with friends and family, lots of travel for me personally enjoying family and a wedding, Colton getting engaged and beginning wedding plans, Brian's continuing neuroscience therapy (at times on a high and encouraged; at times plummeting in frustration), our receiving confirmation about the next steps in life and ministry leading to such excitement and anticipation, then the super hard day having to put down Zeppelin, my beloved dog of ten years (which brings me to tears practically every time I think about it), and also my mother's deteriorating health and coping with that at 1,800 miles away.

I would like to just crawl back under the covers and cry for a few hours or sit and do nothing. But of course I can't. And I have had plethora of times like that coping with life and the stroke effects.

What's the answer? What do I do?

I do shed some tears and then I intentionally think of the blessings and the goodness of God: Brian is doing very, very well! I am really not a caretaker for him anymore, for which I am very grateful! My children are doing well and happy. Colton has found his soulmate and partner for life, and if that was the only reason (which it isn't!) we moved 1,800 miles away, it would've been worth it! I am incredibly blessed with people who are not only my blood relatives, but also some of my favorite people on the planet whom I treasure spending time with. That is a unique joy not everyone can say. My puppy had a wonderful life, was loved, and gave a lot of love. And he is at peace. And I am too. The neuroscience therapy has helped Brian tremendously, and again has proven to be a reason God brought us to Texas. Our needs are met and many of our wants as well. The Lord has been incredibly gracious to us and continues to be an amazing Provider! Just these opportunities to travel have been extraordinary and a blessing. So, I choose life. I choose joy. And that is a choice we all can make each day regardless of circumstances! There is always something to be thankful for. If anyone chooses to put his/her hope in Jesus, then he/she has a Hope that can never be destroyed by circumstances.

See Hebrews 6:18–20 NIV: "We have this hope as an anchor for the soul, firm and secure." Also Psalm 145—we can make a decision to praise.

That writing was interrupted with a call from my friend from here, in fact one of the closest friends I have made in West Texas. She was filling me in on the details of a girl's ranch weekend including a 4-hour trail ride on horseback! (Haha, I am a true novice so will be fodder for amusement I'm sure!) Now this is the real deal! These women are lifetime ranchers/cowgirls/horsewomen—strong, vibrant women here in West Texas. I am honored to be invited! Once again, it was just another reminder of God's timing giving me something fun to look forward to. And that's what I mean—His timing is always perfect. He is so gracious!

April 27, 2015 PRIVATE JOURNAL

While we were driving over to UVA for another sinus checkup, Brian shared that just that morning he had "gotten what he believed was the whole point God wanted to teach him through the stroke in recovery: *Philippians 4:13 NIV, "I can do all things through Christ who strengthens me."* But the point was to realize that verse in the light of verses one through twelve! Brian truly is at peace, more than ever in his life because finally through all of this he has been forced to stop relying on or seeking anything else that signified peace to him. Praise God! I've never seen my husband like this. What a blessing. What an honor to watch. Thank you, Father.

April 29, 2015 Brian: That's the Kingdom of God = peace and rest. I hear so much talk nowadays in Christian circles about "the Kingdom this and the Kingdom that." Frankly, I think much of it is a wrong understanding. Here's what I believe the Kingdom is from my study of Scripture:

The Kingdom is rest, peace, and contentment in whatever God brings into your life. That's why Jesus was able to sleep on the boat in the middle of the storm—because He knew better than anyone on this planet that nothing happens outside God's control. God's plan is unalterable. Nothing happens to me that God doesn't allow or will. Nothing. Satan cannot do anything to me outside of God's sovereign will. I cannot do anything to me outside of God's sovereign will. He knew what I was going to do when He created Adam. Why do I think that I can change it? All I do is accept the ride. I can rest in the back of the boat because I know God has me in His hands. Everything is in His control. I am forever in Him.

Yes, when He taps me and says, "Go over here and do this," I do it. But I am always in His provision. That's what the Kingdom living is— learning to rest and live in that peace and contentment in all things. That's why Paul was able to be all things to all people. That's why Paul was able to sing songs in prison. (Acts 16) That's why Peter was able to go, after he'd been beaten and flogged, into the town center and rejoice that he'd been found worthy to suffer for Christ. (Acts 5) He knew that God is in all things, and that he was in God.

Peter—all the disciples— knew that the Jesus they had walked around with, lived with, ate with, was now with them. That same Spirit now dwelt inside them! They recognized it. Yes, Jesus was their God and their Savior, but He was also their friend. They'd walked around for three years with him. Not only did they witness the incredible miracles and soak in His teaching, they also knew him intimately—heard him belch after supper, seen him when he had to excuse himself to go behind the cactus to relieve himself! I'm not trying to be disrespectful, but I don't think we really. They knew Christ! And they recognized that same Spirit at Pentecost.

That's why they were different. That's why they were so sure of themselves.

When we recognize the fact that it's God Himself now dwelling within us, leading us to a closer walk with Him, guiding us, protecting us, helping us persevere, strengthening us…when we recognize that, how can we not be peaceful in all things? How can we worry about anything? Because the fact is if it doesn't kill me, it makes me stronger. If it kills me, then it takes me to be with Jesus forever. If it doesn't kill me, it's because He still has reason for me to be here. Like Paul said in Philippians 1:21 NIV, *"To live is Christ and to die is gain."*

When you gain that perspective, it's a permanent thing. That's worship! We are to live in that mindset! We are to live in this earth with that perspective. And **that's** the Kingdom come!

GRIEVING THE LOSS
OF THE MUSIC

April 27, 2015

Remember how Brian was talking about Job in the seconds before the stroke began? In the earliest moments of the stroke, I heard the Holy Spirit say to me, "This is a test. It's going to be a hard one, but it's only a test. Brian will be totally healed, totally restored." I have held on to that and believe that means in every way—physically, playing guitar, and spiritually.

We had a visit from a dear friend John yesterday. (He's our drummer for worship band and the one who spent every Sunday morning with Brian while he was in hospital/rehab. They would have bible study together.) Brian was talking about how he can't really play guitar yet and not really sure if God will give that back. I said what I always say: "You need to work at it!" I continued with other advice from a classical musician's perspective—discipline, consistency, effort ... just do it! I also reiterated what I felt the Lord say about him being fully healed.

John had a good word for me, and yes, Lord, I heard You. Perhaps that conviction is just for me to hold in my heart, like Mary "treasuring" ... and leave it between God and Brian. Because it could be that my belaboring that point might actually be hindering the situation instead of enhancing it. Also, John told me that I am not responsible for making that happen. Just let God bring about what He desires. He said it with so much love and respect and I heard Truth.

Thanks, Lord. I want to pray more about that.

*** *Some major truths about this were not realized until February 2016 and following.*

Honestly, the music aspect of this whole journey has been one of the most painful.

Once we got out to Texas, I entered into a time of grieving that I did not expect. Yes, grieving the effects of the stroke in general on my husband, on myself, on every single aspect of our lives together. But also mourning the loss of the music. I only had my electric keyboard with me in Texas and no longer had a private studio space, which were much more significant voids than I anticipated.

For many months I simply did not have the desire in my heart to play. This was a new experience for me. From the time I was a small child, playing the piano and singing had been the deepest and most frequent way I would connect to God. It was a prayer language for me as well as a form of worship, hobby, enjoyment, and vocation.

I had served as a worship leader for over ten years, ministering at various events and retreats as well. During our visit to Fort Davis, Texas, in February 2015 when I asked prayerfully, "What will I do here, Lord?," He had answered in my spirit, "You will worship Me." I, of course, assumed that meant I would be playing and singing a lot. Therefore I really struggled feeling so empty musically. I shared my struggle with my mom June 2016. She admitted great surprise but didn't preach at me, just committed to praying about it.

When I would have time alone and occasionally try to play and sing, I would almost always end up in gut-wrenching weeping. I missed hearing Brian playing guitar, singing, writing music together, having that deep creative bond in private—and public—worship. Since we were eighteen, music was something we had in common. Even when we argued about styles, we still had the music as a unifying force—his background was rock and mine was classical. Try that combination with leading bands and composing songs!

Thankfully, I allowed myself to experience all those feelings honestly. I was not obligated to play or sing anywhere, and I know that was the Lord's mercy for that time.

In the fall 2016, Brian got me a junk baby grand piano, took the keys and hammers out of it, and put my electric keyboard in. Before it was completed, I remember sitting in front of it, gazing at the cavernous hole. And the Lord gave me an object lesson: I, too, had a cavernous hole where the music used to be. In fact, some of the mechanisms that produced the sound had been removed. Eventually, the Spirit got through to me that my music had been "me and God" long before it had ever been "me and Brian." So I went back to music I used to play years ago, rather than trying to do the worship stuff we had so often played together.

Just like that baby grand being given new life, I had to let go of the old in order to embrace the new. Letting go of my acoustic Yamaha P22 (sold it in Virginia instead of moving it) which I had desired for years and had finally purchased felt like losing a part of myself. Not hearing Brian play felt like losing a part of myself. Some of the songs we wrote together are lost because I never played or sang them; only he did. However, my beautiful keyboard—which itself was a gift from God in a great story!—has brought me such joy in the cabinet of a baby grand piano. I have always wanted a grand piano and would not have received it without first letting go. (Come to think of it, I had that Yamaha P22 piano ten years 2005–2015 and I had Zeppelin ten years 2007–2017. Wow.) I had to eventually let go of both. There have been many forms of grief these last few years.

Slowly those wounds began to heal. I also came to the realization that God gave me the talent to play and sing; He made me a worshiper. He has not diminished my gifts at all. Therefore, I must praise Him through music regardless of what Brian does or doesn't do.

April 27, 2015 PUBLIC JOURNAL
Was blessed by this today:

Romans 8:22+. From the Message version

"All around us we observe a pregnant creation. The difficult times of pain throughout the world are simply birth pangs. But it's not only around us; it's within us. The Spirit of God is arousing us within. We're also feeling the birth pangs. These sterile and barren bodies of ours are yearning for full deliverance. That is why waiting does not diminish us, any more than waiting diminishes a pregnant mother. We are enlarged in the waiting. We, of course, don't see what is enlarging us. But the longer we wait, the larger we become, and the more joyful our expectancy.

Meanwhile, the moment we get tired in the waiting, God's Spirit is right alongside helping us along. If we don't know how or what to pray, it doesn't matter. He does our praying in and for us, making prayer out of our wordless sighs, our aching groans. He knows us far better than we know ourselves, knows our pregnant condition, and keeps us present before God. That's why we can be so sure that every detail in our lives of love for God is worked into something good."

A great reminder in this season.

The Lord gave me this song a few years ago. It's entitled HUNGRY and describes the ache in our soul and psyche that can only be filled ultimately when we're present with Christ in Heaven. You can listen for free on our website www.sheilalloydlive.com

Am I hungry for a dinner not yet served on a table not
yet set?

Am I thirsty for a wine that's not been poured for the
bridegroom's not here yet?
People come together, vision has been met
Potential to fulfillment and promises are kept
I'm hungry, I'm hungry for You
I'm thirsty, I'm thirsty for You
I'm waiting, I'm praying for You
Am I seeing a painting not yet made in a color not yet
known?
Am I wanting a mansion not yet built for it needs a living
stone?
A song that won't be sung 'til I join angels 'round the throne
Singing "Holy, Holy" and I'll know that I've come Home
Lord, I'm hungry, I'm hungry for You
I'm thirsty, I'm longing for You
I'm waiting, I'm praying for You

Continuing In
"The Process"

April 28, 2015

Had checkup with sinus doctor at UVA yesterday. Although Brian says he feels great, the doctor says there is still inflammation in his sinuses! So … some different meds. Ninety-minute drive over, sixty-minute wait in waiting room, ten minutes with doctor and how much $? Lol. That's how it goes. It was a gorgeous day, and we had a good lunch in the process.

April 29, 2015

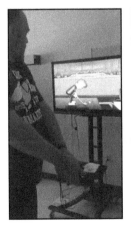 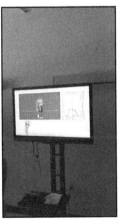

Some fun in therapy!

April 30, 2015

Brian sees a new doctor today...neurologist in Winchester. Pray for insight and wisdom please. Although she doesn't accept our insurance, we believe the Lord directed us to her. She has an excellent reputation and is in frequent communication with his therapist and orthopedist. Thanks for prayers. Appointment is at 10:30 AM.

May 2, 2015

We are putting Colton to work on some Spring projects around the house. He's doing a great job! Took down the ramp, dug out a pathway, and is now putting in stones. Then will paint deck. Gotta say, makes this momma's heart twinge remembering him playing in the dirt pile with cars years ago.

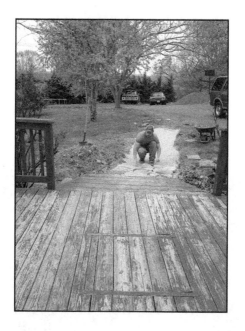

May 7, 2015

FIRST of all, I forgot to post that Brian ran the weed whacker for a while on Saturday! **Yeah**! Stroke in July and weed whacking in May. Only Jesus!

Next, I greatly appreciate it when the Lord uses common—often physical—things to speak to me on a spiritual level. I've been having trouble with my right ear being plugged for the past couple weeks—varying degrees of annoyance, really not pain—despite efforts on my part. What I have learned to do in situations like this is to pray ... not just for the obvious physical healing, but for whatever parallel lessons the Lord might want to teach in the midst of it. I was praying for any obstacles to be removed that were hindering my ability to hear God's voice. I asked that I would hear clearly whatever He wanted me to hear. Finally I went to the doctor this morning. Thankfully, the remedy was a simple cleansing out of impacted earwax (yuck!), apparently a common issue especially with all the pollen. Relief was immediate and drastic, a stark contrast to the "hearing in a barrel" feeling moments before! I was shocked and grateful.

When I left the office I noticed that I was hearing things with sparkling clarity, more than I have noticed in a long time! In fact, the other ear now seemed "dull" compared to the newly cleansed one.

I began to think of the spiritual implications and lessons as I texted my concerned friend, "I am hearing with a clarity and detail that I haven't for a long time!" Hmmmmm ... that'll preach! The remedy to my "hearing loss" was not a complicated one. It didn't take tons of time or cost lots of money. But it required intentionality. Likewise, the remedy to not hearing spiritually requires us to be intentional—make a decision and a commitment to spend time getting to know Jesus' voice through prayer and Bible study. John 10 explains that if we are followers of Jesus—His sheep—then we will hear His voice. Isaiah 30:21 NIV says that we will hear a "still, small voice" whispering behind us. *"Whether you turn to the right or to the left, your ears will hear a voice behind you, saying, 'This is the way; walk in it.'"*

In order to hear, we need to be listening. And in order to listen, our ears need to be clear. Let's allow the Holy Spirit to clear away any obstacles in our lives which hinder our ability to **hear Him** clearly!

May 8, 2015
The new meds from neurologist are kicking his butt!

But the T-shirt over the mouth he has always done. I have no idea why! Lol!

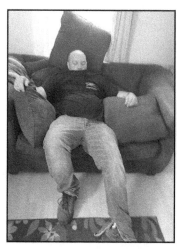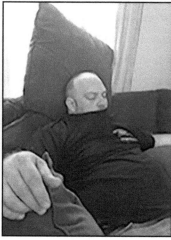

May 8, 2015 PRIVATE JOURNAL:

Besides the issues of Brian's physical challenges during this time, I am also trying to adjust to a different schedule and way of daily life. I was used to having a lot of time alone and really enjoyed it. I like silence and solitude, and the Lord ministered greatly through it. Therefore I am often very frustrated at the lack of quiet and the lack of time alone. One day recently as I walked and prayed, I cried out to the Lord about my longing for solitude. I asked, "What do you want to be to me, Lord?" I heard, "I want to be your schedule, your calendar, your rest."

This season in my life is very different from one year ago. I sense the Holy Spirit wanting to teach me to not lose my joy or my peace when I don't have solitude or when the day doesn't go as I expected. Did Jesus at times long for alone time with the Father, expect it, but then woke up to bickering disciples or an invalid at his feet? Or multitudes requesting bread, both spiritual and physical? And how did he respond? In peace, with love not frustration. Jesus responded with compassion. And yet I don't believe Jesus had any problem with boundaries. He was perfect—fully divine and fully human. (See Hebrews 1:1–3; Colossians 2:9; Isaiah 9:6; John 10:30–39; 14:6-11; Revelation 1:17–18; 22:13)

Yes, at times Jesus called three disciples away with him … to … sit quietly on the beach? Laugh? Pray? Impart? Teach? Rest?

We need rest; we need refreshment. Sometimes physical, frankly always spiritual, and often both! Hebrews 4:1–13 explains that Jesus IS the Sabbath rest. See also Psalm 5:11–12 and Matthew 11:28–30.

We are finite, flawed, physical beings, but we are called to be transformed into his likeness. He does the transforming by the way! See Romans 12:1–2; 2 Corinthians 3:12–18.

What is our part? Surrender and cooperation.

Pictures of various Occupational Therapy sessions and progress. Glory to God! He has worked very hard & these therapists have been wonderful!

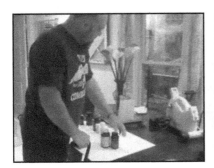
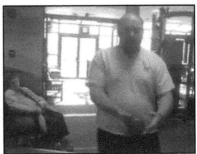
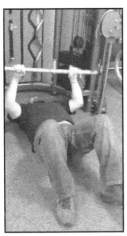
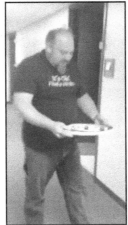
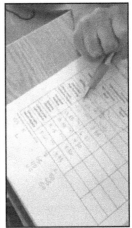

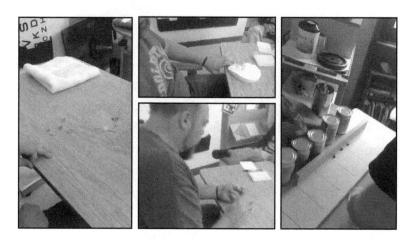

May 11, 2015

We had to wait a couple minutes before therapy today … lol! You therapists must wear people out. **But this is before he started!**

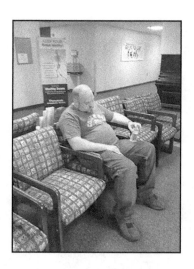

May 12, 2015

Boy, what a difference a few months and good therapists make but mostly the grace and healing of God. Thank you!

May 17, 2015

Brian was discharged from OT by Amy Gray—who we now consider a dear friend!— this past week. She says he has everything he needs at home to continuing working and gaining strength! Yes and thank you, Jesus! We say a deep heartfelt **thank you** to Amy Gray ... has to be the **best** occupational therapist in the Valley! But we might be a teensy bit prejudiced.

May 17, 2015

Brian and I had the privilege this morning to share what the Lord laid on our hearts about worship. It occurred to me as we were getting started that this is the first time publicly since the stroke that we have spoken in front of a group. Isn't it appropriate that the topic was not ourselves or our story **but** rather **Who** God is and why it is appropriate to worship Him!?

Part 2 is next Sunday 10:00 AM. Everyone is welcome— Fresh Water Fellowship, Woodstock, VA. It is being recorded; we do believe this is sign of things to come as far as ministry that we'll be doing together.

May 18, 2015

Micah 7:7 NIV in a card from my mom

"But as for me, I watch in hope for the Lord, I wait for God my Savior; my God will hear me."

*** I remember the day I received that card. Boy, I needed the reminder that I am not hoping or waiting for anything or anyone, just waiting and hoping and trusting in God. So often we feel as though we are waiting for _____ ... you fill in the blank! A baby. A wedding. A date. Healing. A job. A raise. A prodigal child to return home. Recognition. Promotion. Return of joy. When we focus on the _____, we become weary in the waiting. Years ago I learned this and began to see the often quoted scripture Isaiah 40:31 KJV in a different light.

"But they that wait upon the Lord shall renew their strength; they

shall mount up with wings like eagles; they shall run and not be weary; they shall walk and not faint."

*It is, in fact, **in** the waiting—not the achievement—that we mount up and soar! In the waiting—if that waiting is focused on the Lord— that our strength and hope are renewed.*

And the confidence to say "My God will hear me" is truly incredible!

Reflecting and Taking Stock
of Where We Are

*** *I remember vividly writing the journal entry below. It was a gorgeous, sunny, spring day. I sat on the front porch with my dog enjoying the fresh air and beautiful tranquil views. Journaling has always been a cathartic process for me, and I felt the need to spend some time processing the many, many events and emotions.*

May 25, 2015

Wow. One year ago today was a Sunday. Brian and I were in New Castle, Pennsylvania. We had just taken a friend's Mustang back to him (**finally**). Brian had restored it for him from basically the frame, and it had taken years. Because it had unexpectedly taken so long, we had long since spent the client's initial investment. Delivering that car was a **huge** load off us in every way (mentally, financially, and emotionally.) Plus, spiritually we knew that it was an albatross around Brian's neck. He knew that until he did his part and removed it, God could not move us to the next phase that He had planned for us.

While up there, I had a 24-hour getaway mother-daughter time with Mom while Dad was in the Veteran's hospital for respite care. Mom and I had never done anything like that in all my life—gone "just because" to a nice hotel, eaten meals out, went shopping, to the movies, took a

"Duck Boat Tour" of downtown Pittsburgh in reclaimed amphibian vehicles from WWII, and just enjoyed being together. It was a time that I will always treasure!

On Sunday the 25th before heading back to Virginia, Brian and I did Guerrilla Worship in the ravine behind the barn at Eldogor Lane (the property where I grew up which is still family-owned). My niece Carly was there, too. God revealed what/how to pray; Brian played his guitar. I moved out first since I had the most tie and call (and therefore spiritual authority) to the land. It was a very significant time to me emotionally and spiritually.

On our way back to Virginia, we stopped and visited Dad at the Veteran's facility in Butler. It was heart-wrenching and yet wonderful to sit with him and some other men as they shared their stories from WWII.

The weekend was truly a highlight to me for so many reasons, not the least of which was that Brian and I had such a good time together on the trip. We listened to the Jason Upton CD "Open Up the Earth" the whole drive up. The entire weekend was bathed in God's Presence.

Since that weekend, **so** much life has happened! My last visit with Dad was on July 4. Brian had the stroke July 10. Dad died August 2. I became a caretaker of my husband as well as Garrett. Colton truly stepped up to the plate responsibility-wise, and my daily rhythm of life was drastically altered. God has taught me **so** much, for which I am deeply grateful! Yet I admit that for the last couple weeks I have been tired again, weary of the process, wishing for the end of this life season, praying to hold on to the faith and belief for the promise of "full healing/ full restoration" that I really believe the Lord gave me in the first hours after the stroke.

It is again Memorial Day weekend, and the weather could not be more perfect. Zeppelin and I walked this morning down our beautiful lane as I prayed out loud and poured out my heart to the Father. My flesh is weary. I'm tired of my husband being "less than" physically. Even our intimate life together is compromised, and that is a problem we have never had in almost twenty-five years of marriage. Brian has often said over these last few months that it seems like the Lord has taken everything away from him—everything that made him "him," defined him, gave him a sense of strength and identity. He recognizes that God's purpose is that Brian find his **total** identity in the Lord. And although that is an incredible blessing to hear one's husband say, the walking through it is not easy.

Hidden in an alcove of trees, I prayerfully knelt to the ground in tears, "Abba, Father!" After a few seconds I listened to nature around me—birds' songs, whistling insects, and the whooshing wind in the tops of the trees. The Holy Spirit brought to mind several things: the Lord watches over every sparrow, and He has promised to watch over me as well. He sees me. He is aware of what is happening in my life, and He knows my struggle with it. The wind in the tops of the trees reminded me of the passage in 2 Samuel 5:22–25 where God uses that as a sign to David that He will make him victorious in battle. It was a reminder of His Presence. Thank you, Lord.

A few weeks ago on the drive to UVA for the checkup with sinus surgeon (and there is still inflammation!) Brian commented that he felt more at peace than he ever has in his whole life! He shared that every day, he wakes up and truly feels deep peace. He says it is almost a euphoric feeling, and he knows it is Christ's peace. (John 14:26–27) Wow! Brian says that he worked from the time he was fifteen years old, so all he's ever known is to get up and go to work. Although he was hearing the Lord's call to a radically different way of life and into full-time ministry, he could not rationally make that switch in his head. He didn't know **how** to go about surrendering that aspect of himself and making alternative choices. Well, the stroke took care of that.

Around 9:30 PM Thursday July 10, 2014, his way of life was radically altered! Brian says that he does not believe that God "caused" the stroke. However, he does believe that God allowed it. The lessons he—and all of us—have learned could not have been learned otherwise. We now have experienced living truly by the grace of God. Brian prayed in the ambulance, "Okay, Lord, if you want to bring me home to Heaven now, that's fine. I'm ready to be with you. If you have more you want me to do here, then let me live. Whatever You want is fine with me." He says when he woke up in ICU the next morning, he figured, "Guess God has more plans for me here. Okay then."

May 25, 2015 Brian: letting go of life/job/passion
In August 2013 we went out for a trip to Fort Davis, Texas, when I was working and physically fine. That's when we both felt called to move there. To leave behind us the life we had built. We talked about it. It's easy to think about that in your head. But physically, I didn't know how to let go. I loved what I did, where I worked. It was a dream job. It was a job that, when I took it, I thought I'd be there until I died or the owner died. Haha. It was one of those jobs encapsulating what I'd been striving for my whole life.

It was hard for me to let that go. I just didn't know how. I had built up cars, mechanics and restoration in my head for so long that those pursuits became *who* I was. Even though God had gotten me out of the box playing music, which had actually become much more important to me than the car world, I still could not figure out in my mind how to make the switch from doing life the way I always had. It's as if God was saying, "I know. And I know what's coming that will help you make that switch—will make the transition for you."

So when I suffered the stroke, that old identity stripped itself away. It wasn't something that I had to do, explain to all my friends, constantly fight the desire to get back involved. No. It was just BANG! Overnight I was done. Cold turkey.

Sheila: I remember your saying to me—with very slow, slurred speech—in ICU probably less than 24 hours after the stroke hit, "I think the Ferrari gig is up."

Brian: Yes, you know, even though I still retain everything I knew about cars—I still have a lot of knowledge and a lot to offer as far as that goes—but I knew immediately that gig was done. I couldn't go back. Even if God restored me physically, I realized at that point that part of my life was gone.

Sheila: It's like the apostle Peter going back to fishing after Jesus was crucified.

Brian: Yes. Even if God has me do something with cars again, it's not going to be the same. It's not going to be the same thing. I don't know how to explain it better than that. You have to be stripped away to understand that the identity you make for yourself, build or fashion for yourself, is not who you are. Your identity in Christ is what's real. That's what you depend on. That's what you trust, what you live by. And that's a different way of thinking! In this new mindset, you just let it go and let God. I know that's a very trite saying; it's been so overused. But it's true. At the core of what it means, it's true. You let go and learn to listen to God. Learn to listen to that still small voice…because He wants to just nudge you, not hit you over the head with a two by four like He had to with me.

Sheila PRIVATE JOURNAL continued May 25, 2015
We have learned the true meaning of relying on God's provision. He is our Provider, not Brian's income, not mine, not the government programs, not Disability money, not food stamps. Now the Lord often uses all of those means, but He is the Source. We have lived ten-and-half months now under a budget that makes no sense on paper. Kingdom math is different. And we have not lacked for one thing we have needed! Actually, even many of our wants have been supplied! Praise You, Lord!

A question I learned to ask early on (through a sermon on CD) is, *"Lord, what do you want to **be** for me right now that you could not be at any other time?"* Those answers have been poignant and fascinating, each one timely and revelatory to the moment I asked. Answers like,

"Your Rock, Strength, Peace, Provision, teaching you how to love and how to serve as I served you, your Refuge, your Joy" among others.

Because of this experience, the Lord is preparing us to take the next huge step of faith—to uproot our family and move across the country, to begin a life of full-time ministry which will likely look quite different from the world's or even the Church's definition of "normal"!

The way of life that we have established and operated under for the last twenty-plus years has been turned upside down. And although that turning has been challenging—and we do grieve the loss at times—in actuality that turning is providing a **freedom** and a peace we would never have expected. We have had an opportunity during this season to learn radical dependence on God, a faith that is not based on popular opinion or data but rather on that still small Voice spoken in our hearts through the Holy Spirit. We have seen the Lord bringing to pass the wealth of the wicked being stored up and transferred to the righteous. (Proverbs 13:22 and Ecclesiastes 2:26) Fascinating lessons. Life-changing realizations.

I needed to write today. Thank you, Lord, for the perspective that You bring to me when I process with You.

Brian says the most difficult part of the stroke for him is not being able to play guitar. That has hit him in a very deep place emotionally, as playing guitar has always been a huge part of who he is. It also has been the main way that he prays and worships. He has commented that playing is like his speaking in tongues. The classically trained teacher/ musician in me steps in and says, "Well, you just need to force yourself to practice 15 minutes every day. Just do it and it will get better. Maybe God is wanting you to take that step and put forth the effort and discipline before He will give it back."

His not being able to play has affected me deeply as well. Playing music together while leading worship was a way that we connected on a deeply spiritual level. I heard the anointing in his playing, and I desperately miss it. Since I have still been leading the worship team at church through this time, his absence changed the makeup of our team. There are songs we can't do without him, because he played and sang lead. He hasn't really been able to sing since the stroke either (and I'm sure the sinus junk didn't help).

Thanksgiving Day was the first time he tried to play the guitar in front of me since the stroke. It was just a few notes and sounded like a beginner's "picking" but it was sweet music to my ears! In January he started playing bass with the team. He's never considered himself a bass player, and it is not his instrument of choice. But it is a way he can be back up with us leading worship, and he feels it is what the Lord wants him to do right now. He says it is getting slightly easier, but playing requires a ton of concentration just to play each note. He has to "tell" his fingers every little motion. But as far as the guitar, he doesn't try to play it very much... says it's too emotionally difficult. I cannot imagine how frustrating it would be to sit at the piano, knowing everything in my mind but not being able to make my fingers do it! Heart-wrenching to be sure!

I'll admit, though, I have gotten very frustrated and even angry with him because in my judgement (and therein lies the problem), he wasn't trying hard enough, doing enough, believing enough, exercising faith that Jesus would heal him. After all, doesn't he remember that God told him he would be restored? I know I heard from the Lord in the first moments of the stroke while in our studio, "This is a test, guys. It's a big one, but it's a test. He will be fully healed and fully restored." I am not a name-it, claim-it person, but I do believe I heard this.

While Brian was in the hospital, God would wake me in the mornings and the initial thought in my mind would be a specific thing to pray for Brian that day. Sometimes it was physical, most often spiritual. And so that would begin my day and my exercise of belief. Perhaps I need to ask the Lord to do that again—yes, please, Lord. I do believe; help my unbelief. (Mark 9:24) When time marches on and we don't see the total healing—the way we define it and expect it!— we begin to wonder if we heard correctly. I do not want to be tossed by waves of doubt (James 1:2–8) Please write on my heart Your word, Your promise.

At any rate, a few weeks ago a dear friend of ours (fellow musician) visited us at home. He spent the afternoon mostly chatting with Brian about the Word, the Lord, and various life stuff. (This was the same friend who spent Sunday mornings with Brian in the hospital having church together instead of coming and playing on the worship team with us. Perhaps part of that was it was just too hard to play without Brian there. I understand.) We sat at dinner that evening and he asked Brian about playing guitar—how was it coming? Brian shared the process and the challenges physically as well as emotionally. I interjected my perspective. At that point the Lord spoke through our friend to me in a powerful (and yet very loving and gracious way). I'll paraphrase what he said. "Sheila, that's great if that's what you heard the Lord say. Hang on to that. But perhaps in this case what you need to do is to store that up in your heart like Mary did about Jesus (Luke 2:19). You don't need to say anything to Brian or to others. Let that be between you and the Lord. And let Brian's journey with playing again be between him and the Lord. You are not responsible for him in this." So true! Thank you, Lord.

As I have prayed about that since, I needed to confess that I was trying to control things. I was feeling like I had to convince Brian (and other people) of what I heard the Lord say in order for it to come to pass. Like I had a responsibility to do first that would free God to act. Forgive my arrogance, Lord! I wanted to ease my pain. I wanted to ease his pain. But that is not in my control, and it is not my responsibility. A close girlfriend and fellow musician did encourage me, though, that I need to stand in the gap and believe for him in that matter until he has the strength to believe it himself.

Since that day we have talked about guitar very little. His OT asked him frequently and tried to encourage him saying similar things that I had said. I know it still rips into his heart, and yet he has also expressed that incredible sense of peace in Christ.

Yesterday while driving to church in the morning—and we were preaching on worship for the second week—Brian said the Lord had told him something: he needs to focus on walking right. (The left foot, stepping correctly, and walking smoothly is still a big challenge. When we had prayed together in early April, God had revealed the dual learning point of walking physically and walking spiritually. It was after that time of prayer that he got his brace adjusted, started seeing a new PT, and changed to an excellent neurologist.) Back to yesterday—he said God told him when he got the walk figured out, then the Lord would give back the music. He needs to have his spiritual walk right first because God is going to teach him how to play where it is totally Truth. It won't be his flesh at all. Praise You, Lord! Thank you for that word and that encouragement! We trust You.

I am **choosing** by an act of the will and obedience—because it is not in my emotions lately—to give **praise** and to be thankful, listing out specific things. Besides the many things I've listed in the preceding paragraphs, I think back in my mind to the physical journey since July 10. **Huge** recovery.

PRAISE YOU, JESUS!

A SIGNIFICANT CHOICE

May 26, 2015 PUBLIC JOURNAL

Although we have **so** much to be thankful for these last ten-and-a-half months, at times we still have bouts of discouragement. Appreciate your prayers. Thanks.

May 28, 2015 PUBLIC JOURNAL

The last few days I have had more times of thinking, "This is not what I planned... I'm tired of the challenges in this season... I'm ready to see that complete healing...." So I have deliberately chosen to praise God, like the Psalmist did.

This morning, though, I was reminded that Jesus said, *"In this world you will have trouble; but take heart, I have overcome the world!"* (John 16:33 NIV)

Many of us are facing circumstances in our lives that are less than ideal... health struggles, financial difficulties, a broken marriage, a sick child... well, it's true—life is hard, **but God is Good**!

May we **choose to** put our whole hope, emphasis, and trust in God Most High and our loving Lord Jesus. He is the only true Hope, and He has **overcome**! When I am weak, then I am strong in Him, then his power is manifest in me. 2 Corinthians 12:9–10. A humbling and challenging reminder.

May 30, 2015

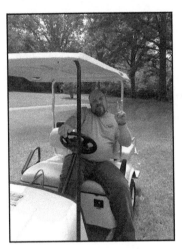

We are in Pennsylvania at Eldogor Lane celebrating my niece's wedding this weekend (today). Eldogor Lane has been the family homestead since my dad designed and built it in 1957. It is truly one of my favorite places on the planet and one that, by God's grace, has always exuded peace, security and love, not to mention incredible beauty of surrounding nature—huge oak trees, woods, ravine, stream, and random wildlife. It's great to see Brian getting around driving golf carts, holding flashlights, offering the car hood for my dear brother, father of the bride, to stand on top of in order to repaint the basketball hoop and backboard.

Not only a beautiful wedding, but poignant celebration of family and faith on this beloved property. Treasured memories!

June 2, 2015 Facebook post

Most of you know that we went back to New Castle, Pennsylvannia, this past weekend to help out and then enjoy the beautiful outdoor family wedding of my niece Dawn. Besides the heart-warming laughter, jokes, food, etc. that comes along with being with my great family, I learned some other things as well.

As I shared last week, we have been a little discouraged lately. It's been a rough almost eleven months. So the time away was a blessing to focus on something different, be around so many wonderful people, friends new and old.

But here's what I realized: everyone goes through hard times. Some glimpses of challenges that I was exposed to in the lives of people these past 72 hours:

* ongoing chronic pain
* a child with multiple physical challenges but a very bright mind, rolling around in a walker—even down the wedding aisle throwing rose petals
* a man who went through cancer in his thirties as his wife and young children watched
* many people who had gone through some form of cancer
* a thirteen-year-old severely mentally and physically disabled young man who sat contentedly for several hours while his parents visited with friends.
* a man recovered from open heart triple bypass surgery and one who'd had a heart transplant
* someone who's had a couple hip replacements
* people with financial challenges
* a woman trying to escape the emotionally draining continuing drama of family members
* a mother whose son is incarcerated

The list goes on....

Do you understand my point? I guess what I realized is that we **all** face trials. Again, Jesus said, *"In this world you **will** have trials."*

Yes, we have been through a tough time this year. Yes, we get weary. But we are not alone. I think part of the importance of community and fellowship is that we **encourage** one another as we travel this path called **life**. The conclusion of Jesus' statement I mentioned above was, *"**But** take heart, I have overcome the world!"* (John 16:33 NIV)

Joy of wedding plans, smiles, laughter, being creative, digging around the barn for clever rustic décor, great food, new friends, renewing old friendships, playing music, hearing a fresh perspective on marriage vows, being **thankful** for **so** many blessings ... my heart is refreshed; my soul is revived. Thank you, Lord. I can continue on the journey because of **You**.

LOOKING AHEAD

*** *A letter to close family written in June 2015. Looking back, I think I was seeking approval in some ways, for which I repented for later. The only approval we need is from the Lord. However, we have always been very close to our families and wanted to share what was going on.*

Hope you guys are doing well! We are getting along fine, settling into summer.

I think you are aware that God is calling us to move to Fort Davis, Texas, for ministry. This is something that has been building since the summer of 2012. We prayerfully continued to seek Him as we traveled there in August 2013, and at that point were convinced it was indeed the next step. We were getting ready to put the house on the market last summer before Brian had the stroke. Obviously, every aspect of our lives has been turned upside down, so we weren't sure exactly how the next steps would unfold. However, this last eleven months have only served to further clarify our conviction, willingness, and excitement to step into this new venture! And this time has certainly deepened our faith and confidence that the Lord will provide! If He can do everything He's done physically, spiritually, and financially through all this, then He can certainly guide our steps and make provision for us moving across the country!

Our trip out there in February 2015 was kind of "Lord, has anything changed, or is this indeed what you want us to pursue?" I sensed in my spirit (although He doesn't mind our asking for confirmation), "Yes! And if you continue to ask, you will be walking in disobedience."

Please, keep us in prayer!

This spring, we did a few things around the house which needed to be addressed. Then I asked a realtor friend for some advice. She came up with another long list of things to do before officially putting it on the market. We started to get bids, etc. but then were convicted last week—if God said to go, then put it on the market now. Let Him deal with it! I put it on Craigslist Monday night and got two calls by Thursday noon. We'll see. We trust it to the Lord's hands completely. We surrender to His timing.

Although we love our life here and have wonderful friendships, we do sense that the Lord has "lifted our calling" for the Valley. It's been eighteen-and-a-half years here. In fact in the last few months we have watched the Lord kind of separating relationships (not at all in a negative way) as word got around that we were sensing a move. We have prayed together for the Lord to put people in our paths while we are still here and use this remaining time for His purposes. And indeed, it has been really cool to watch what has developed after that prayer!

Obviously the biggest things on my heart about this big of a move is the boys and my mom. Colton is twenty. He plans to stay for a while here with Brian's parents, but knows that eventually he will be in Texas with us. Garrett is technically a senior this fall, but he can stay in school until he's twenty-one since he has an IEP. Fort Davis is a small close-knit town, and the reputation of the special education there is very good. We see that school would be a good way for him—and all of us— to make inroads into the community.

I certainly do not relish being further away from my mom. But she has known of our calling for a couple years now. Her response is one I greatly admire and respect: "Honey, you have to do what God tells you to do! I will be OK." Gordon and Lois have certainly been very good to her! She also has commented many times in the last few months how blessed she is with some very good friends in New Castle. Besides being kind and helpful to her (especially during these last several months), they genuinely enjoy her company, provide encouragement, laughter and camaraderie. It blessed me, and I have thanked them. **You** all also have been so wonderful to her, for which I am truly grateful! I am believing and trusting that I will get to go home to visit her a few times a year. I have to trust the Lord that He loves Mom more than I do and will provide for her needs in every way whether I am physically present or not.

God has made clear to us that this process will be somewhat like Abraham when God told him to leave everything and **go** to a land He would show to him. In the going, the details will become clearer. (Genesis 12)

This has truly been an interesting process, being raised in a missionary family and hearing these types of testimonies. Never before have I really experienced it myself. I have more compassion and insight into the challenges and joys that my grandparents and other family have faced! **But God** ... we have no choice but to obey in light of His faithfulness and love.

We do not know the timing of events. When God sells the house, we can go.

Thank you for joining with us in prayer!

HIS on the Adventure,
Sheila

Isaiah 42:16

Continuing "The Process" Physically and Spiritually

June 10, 2015

Please continue to pray for Brian's recovery. The main issue right now is still that left foot. We need to have another consult with the lady who made the brace and also check in with PT. He can lock his knee in and walk pretty quickly, but that makes his knee really sore. He's been being very deliberate on how he places his left foot—to walk without snapping the knee. But walking that way makes his right hip sore because of all the overcompensation. It's frustrating.

On the positive side, though—turning this challenge into a prayer: he's been praying that the Lord would teach him a new way to **walk** (physically **and** spiritually). In light of that, we began a Word study today.

Brian truly senses that this "walk" is the crux of the matter right now.

Wow. Just realized today is the tenth. Eleven months today. Ugh. I'd be lying if I said I didn't just want him to be physically **all better** now. **But** again, the lessons we have learned this past year spiritually are priceless. So I say, "Thank You, Lord. I trust You." Give us strength in Jesus' name.

June 10, 2015 Brian: walking

About walking…. Physically, I look at walking. It's something we take for granted! You don't think about how you walk—how you stride, how you move you leg, foot, ankle, and hip in order to walk. I was trying to learn to walk without my knees locking or hyperextending, so I was evaluating my walk constantly. I was also always watching and evaluating how everyone around me was walking. If you had to sit and think about how to take a step, would you know how to make your leg do it?

Sheila: No.

Brian: No. You just know how to do it! I'm trying to think about, "Okay, do I move my hip first or my knee? When do I start to bend my knee? What are my toes supposed to be doing? What about my ankle? What is it supposed to do?"

It's strange how I was thinking about it! I had to be very intentional.

And now I see where God has brought me, compared to where I was. Even towards the end of the first year after the stroke, although I was able to walk around, I was still very unstable, wobbly, very straight-legged. Now I evaluate how I'm walking—even though I'm not where I want to be, it's amazing how much better I am! I can walk farther, longer, and with more stamina.

Isn't that very spiritual? We're not where we want to be, but we can look back from where God has brought us. I'm again reminded of Philippians, where it says, *"Offer up your prayers and supplication to the Lord with a thankful heart, giving thanks for what He has done."* (Philippians 4:6 NKJV, *my paraphrase*) We offer our requests up to God. I pray all the time still, "God, heal me. Jesus, heal me. Lord, heal me. Restore me to what I was. Lift me up." But also, I thank Him for where He has brought me! He has not abandoned me. He has not neglected me. He has not left me alone. I give God thanks for all the things He has given me back. It's a "now but not yet" kind of thing. He has healed me. He is healing me, and He will heal me. He has saved me. He is saving me, and He will save me. When we are in Christ, we are in a constant renewing, constant growing. It's a process. It's ongoing.

Sheila: That's the transformation. (2 Corinthians 3:12–18)

Brian: Until the day we meet Him face to face. When we see Him face to face, finally the transformation will be complete; and we will know all the secrets, all the mysteries of Heaven. Until then, we learn them a little bit at a time, so that we're never quite there but we're a lot farther along than we used to be.

June 12, 2015

Remember the $41,000 helicopter ride Brian took from Winchester ER up to Fairfax INOVA the night of the stroke? Well.....after months and months, Anthem still has only agreed to pay $7,000 toward that bill. We—well, actually our unpaid but highly valued "secretary" Aimee Patrick has the commissioner of insurance (or some such title) involved, but it looks as though it is coming to the end of what they can do. PHI Medical (who flew) are appealing one more time I believe.

As of yet we have not been billed for the $34K-plus balance.

We are praying and trusting the Lord to work it out. Thanks for joining us in that.

June 12, 2015

At Bible study last night I was struck with three little words, "Come and see."

We were studying John chapter 1. In 1:35–39, a couple of his first disciples set out to follow him. They asked Jesus where he was staying. Apparently, this was more than just a "In what hotel are you staying?" type of question. It is more of a declaration that they wanted to be trained by him.

Jesus' response was, "Come and you will see."

That stopped me in my tracks. Such a simple answer. Such a clear directive. You want to know me, want to know what I'm about? Come and you will see.

Jesus gave no fanfare, made no hype. Didn't even do any miracles right then (that we know of). He just said, "Come and see." This was the Lord God Almighty in the flesh, the Word who spoke creation into existence. I can picture the scene in my mind. John 1:38 NIV says, *"Turning around Jesus saw them following and asked, 'What do you want?'"* I can imagine Jesus, upon hearing their answer, casually turning back around and calmly saying, *"Come and you will see."*

What questions arise in your mind about Jesus? What are the things you feel you need to know about life, about Christianity, about death? Truth is found in only one place. Jesus said in John 14:6 NIV, *"I am the Way. I am the Truth. I am the life. No one comes to the Father except by me."* So instead of exhausting yourself chasing everything under the sun and trying to avoid those questions, perhaps you should just follow Jesus' advice—"Come and you will see."

Take the risk. Test Him out. What do you have to lose? What might you have to gain? Jesus either was who he said he was … or he was a raving lunatic! There is no in between. There is no "He was a good teacher." But decide for yourself…

Come and you will see.

If you would like someone to talk to or help you begin that journey, I would count it a supreme privilege!

June 14, 2015

"You will keep in perfect peace him whose mind is steadfast because he trusts in you. Trust in The Lord for he is the Rock Eternal!" Isaiah 26:3–4 NIV

We have to fix our mind but then the Lord gives and sustains the peace!

June 18, 2015

> *"Bless the Lord O my soul! All that is within me bless his holy name. Bless the Lord O my soul! And forget not all his benefits. He forgives all my sins, heals all my diseases, redeems my life from the pit, and crowns me with love and compassion. He satisfies my desires with good things, so that my youth is renewed like the eagles. Bless the Lord O my soul!" Psalm 103:1–5 NIV*

June 20, 2015
My three men are at a car show…
This is my happy place!

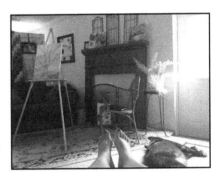

June 23, 2015
Negotiating with creditors … appreciate prayer. We have continued to see the Lord's favor, for which we are truly grateful!

June 24, 2015
Went to PT today for the first time in a long time. You know when you're in a journey of long recovery when your therapist become your friends! They were encouraging to Brian and helpful as always.

We truly are grateful for the folks God has put in our path these last eleven months! I don't know if they realize what an encouragement they are. Today the PT said that Brian is doing so well, that he has made such a great recovery **and** continues to show progress. Most of the time insurance stops paying or the clients get frustrated and stop coming to therapy. It's exciting for her to see someone this long after the stroke.

Just a couple more examples of the Lord's faithfulness.

June 26, 2015

One year stroke anniversary—gotta think of a better name—coming up July 10. Hard to believe! What a year! Challenges and blessings.

We are taking a friend's recommendation to do something special to celebrate and give thanks for all God's done and for more time here together. Thinking of an overnight in Lexington, Virginia... suggestions? (I put this shout out on Facebook and got plenty!)

One thing I'd like to look at is a jeweler who can custom-design rings. I lost a diamond out of my wedding ring last fall. Since we will celebrate twenty-five years in December, Brian says it's time for a new one! Would like to use the remaining diamonds... (I did not end up doing this. By the time I got it repaired, I was so happy to see it on my finger again! I didn't want to change it. Brian says I have nine other fingers that he can put some diamonds on! I said, "Sounds good to me.")

*** *Looking back as we approached the one-year anniversary of the stroke, I remember having such mixed feelings about it. In many ways it was just surreal. Certainly it was never something I had thought about in my wildest imagination. I was angry about it in a sense—thought the Lord would've brought the total healing by this point, didn't want this to be the reality of our lives. On the other hand, certainly I was grateful Brian was still alive and by my side! And of course, could not deny the incredible life lessons and character development, not to mention marriage enrichment and spiritual growth we had experienced over the last year.... All reasons to be grateful. But again, some days I had to make a definite decision for a positive perspective. Isn't that true for all of us so often in life?!*

June 29, 2015 From my note to a friend:

It is going very well with Mac here (the homeless man we met at FWF and God laid it on Brian's heart to have him stay.) Truly, much better than I anticipated. (Guess that's because God set it up!) Our time together Wednesday morning, especially the prayers, really touched him. We have watched him "come alive" over the past week as he volunteers to help with projects around here. Remember how Brian made the comment about not being able to do the weed whacker? After you guys left and without any prompting, Mac went and got the weed whacker from the garage. Over the course of the day, he did practically our whole yard including the big banks in front! What a blessing! Then yesterday he painted the trim on our garage doors. The Lord has really given us perspective through having him here, and it has been enjoyable. God just continues to amaze us.

*** *Yes! You read that correctly. In the middle of putting our house on the market and continuing recovery from the stroke, Brian felt led to have a homeless man stay at our house for a couple weeks. I remember the evening I came in from teaching in the studio and Brian posed that question to me. Everything inside me wanted to yell, "No!" Actually I wanted to yell, "Have you lost your mind? No!" However, I had a strong urging of "What would Jesus do?" And so I said, "Yes." Now Brian used wisdom and caution, laid down some ground rules, and we welcomed Mac into our home. Turned out to be a huge blessing to him and to us and he remains a dear friend to this day, although we haven't been able to get in touch with him the last few months.*

Remember about the credit cards? VISA settled with us for 40 percent of the debt. Turned out we were able to withdraw some $ from a life insurance policy with no penalty! We had never thought of that! I tried to call Discover once I had the $. They were not willing to negotiate at all! Brian heard in his spirit while I was talking with them, "Well, we tried to do everything honestly while being proactive. If they're not willing to work with us, then they are not getting anything." He sensed that the Lord had just settled all our debt. Thank you, Jesus!!

The helicopter bill is still outstanding at $34K-plus and a couple other smaller ones. I have a couple more sets of financial aid paperwork to fill out. Honestly, we are not concerned! God has proven Himself **so** faithful!

July 2, 2015

On my way alone to see my mom for a couple days and attend the Mooney reunion! I forgot how much traffic there is in Berkeley Springs, West Virginia on a holiday weekend. I've been sitting in traffic for 15 minutes in a mile-long line of cars going 5 miles an hour.

Blessings to focus on during this time: solitude. It's not too hot so I can have the windows down; quiet—except for all the cars going by the other way—time to think, time to pray, time to worship.

July 7, 2015

A new "normal"… more on that later.

*** *That was a difficult pill to swallow! Continues to be difficult to grasp … even three-plus years later at this writing.* **I remember a similar struggle after Garrett was born and diagnosed with Down's Syndrome. At a women's conference I heard Barbara Johnson make the statement, "Normal is just a setting on your dryer!" She was a very funny and yet poignant speaker; this statement helped me to take steps toward acceptance and finding joy in an extremely new journey. Same with the stroke. We can spend precious energy and time longing, pining, and whining for the "way things used to be." The truth is, life has changed. There is no way we can go back, BUT there are MANY elements of JOY in this new journey! If we fix our eyes on Jesus, the Author and Perfector of our faith, then we can move into the future with His strength and perspective.**

July 9, 2015

There are many thoughts swirling in my mind today. Tomorrow will be **one year**! Hard to believe it! We are incredibly **thankful** for Brian still being with us and for how **much** strength and mobility he has regained. Glory to God!

In the midst of that, though, there are realities of current challenges. He was telling me this morning, "You and everyone think

I'm fine. Even my therapist told me if she didn't know me she wouldn't know I'd had a stroke. And I am doing well. But you don't realize that I have to concentrate on every single detail, telling my body to do every single individual move. For me just to 'go get a cup' involves dozens of individual steps for my brain to tell my body to do that. I get tired quickly, mentally and physically."

Please continue to pray for Brian's commitment to daily workouts and just tenacity.

July 9, 2015 BRIAN … STEPS TO GET A CUP
I had to think about all these processes in order to do a simple movement physically. For example, to get up from the table, walk across the kitchen, and get a glass out of the cupboard, here are the steps I had to go through mentally in order to accomplish that simple task:

Okay, stand up. Put weight on foot. Stand up. Push with my calf and ankle. Bend the knee. Support with the hip and thigh. Take a step. And another and another until I get over to the cupboard. Oh, now open the cupboard door with my left hand. Grab the cup. Grasp the cup. Pull it out. Keep holding onto the cup. Don't let the cup drop. Walk back to the table carrying the cup. Sit back down. And this was intensified if there was actually liquid **in** the cup!

All these things that your brain has to do!

Sheila: Truly amazing.

Brian: Yes, amazing that my brain did it without my even thinking about it before! What I have found is that when I go through times of exhaustion—physically and mentally—is also when I notice huge gains shortly afterwards. Something was regenerating in my body, so my brain was working overtime. I would go through times when I was really exhausted and would sleep a lot. It was as though my brain was rebooting or working harder than normal, so it was making me more tired. If that makes any sense. That's what I've noticed. Therefore, I've come to appreciate those times when I'm really tired because I think, "Aha! Something's getting ready to happen!"

Sheila: That'll preach!

Brian: Think about that spiritually for a while: you come to appreciate those times when you're feeling really exhausted because you know that something is getting ready to happen. I won't say anything more about that. You just think about that for a while.

Sheila's journal continued:
Please pray that I would be strengthened by Jesus' love and ability to serve... helping when Brian needs me but not hovering... and some opportunities for rest and solitude for myself too.

We're going to go out of town Friday–Saturday just to be together, **celebrate** and praise!

ONE YEAR ANNIVERSARY
OF THE STROKE

July 10, 2015

Brian and I went away just to praise and celebrate everything God has done this past year. Went to Lexington, Virginia. Most of the time was just spent driving (beautiful scenery and weather) and talking, reflecting, and anticipating what is ahead with move to Fort Davis, Texas. We drove from Lexington down to Hot Springs, Virginia, where we had honeymooned almost twenty-five years ago.

Lying in the hotel room on the morning of July 11, I got kind of emotional... last July 11 waking up in a hotel room without him and my whole world was turning upside down. He held me close and said, "Sheila, you are an amazing woman! We both stood strong in the Lord and just took the challenge of the enemy. And I believe God is going to reward us for that stance and our faith in Him. This coming year is going to be very interesting!"

July 11, 2015

Time together around Lexington and Hot Springs, VA

We were in Hot Springs, Virginia, on our honeymoon too!

From a video Brian made sitting on a stone wall overlooking a beautiful valley and river near Lexington, Virginia, July 11, 2015.

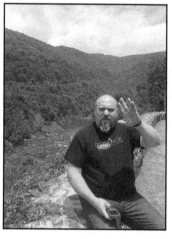

Hey, everybody! We're out here in this beautiful part of the country celebrating a year of "new life" so to speak! As I've been on this year's journey of recovery, I've had to ask myself time and time again "Lord, what did You want to show me through this? What have You wanted me to learn? I don't think You caused the stroke, but there is something You're showing me in this. Otherwise, why did you save me from the stroke?"

I think one of the things I've learned is that there is the absolute truth of the Word of God. That means I read the Bible. I don't interpret the Bible in light of what I want it to say. There are things it says that I must admit are true—whether I like them or not. There are things we do or don't do—not because that is how we earn our salvation, but because simply because that's the way God did it. He's God, and He has the right to do things any way He wants to because He's God! I don't have the right to ask Him why He establishes truth the way He does. It's a hard lesson! There are plenty of things in my own life He's shown me that I just can't continue to do. I've got to have the faith to hand them over to Christ and say, "Your way is better than mine."

I'm not just talking about the recent hubbub [the ruling on homosexual marriage]— honestly, who thought it would go any differently than it did? But it's more than that. That's one example. The fear of God means that we don't do the things He doesn't like and we do do the things He does!

Honestly, why do we accept Christ? Is it just because we're afraid of going to hell? Why do I accept Christ as my Savior?

Because without Him in my life, without believing that He is the only truth, the Son of God who came and died for my sins and raised from the dead—if I don't believe those things, then the Bible is very clear that I am going to hell. We have to accept the Bible as Absolute Truth. The reason our culture is in the mess that it's in is because we want to erode Absolute Truth. We want to try to interpret morality with our eye on what we want it to say, what we think is fair, what we think is right. It doesn't matter what we think is right or fair. What matters is what we know God said is right, just, or fair. There's a difference.

Maybe I'm not real clear on this. I'm still trying to wrap my head around it, because God is revealing things to me through this process as I study and as I walk and learn. It's hard, and I'd be glad to talk with anybody who wants to talk about it, whether in discourse or even debate.

It simply comes down to this: do you believe God is real and therefore true and honest in what He says? Either He is or He isn't. God isn't messing around. He's not just playing. If we don't follow Him, we have no hope. I'm sorry if you disagree with me. You have the right to follow your own path, but you also have the right to one day face the consequences of not following God if that's what you choose. Because there is a God, only one God, and it's the God in the Bible. It's not the god in the Quran. He's not the god of the Buddhists nor is He one of the many gods of the Hindus. He's not the god of the Jehovah Witnesses. He's also not the god of the Mormons—that's a different god. The Bible says if you hear a different gospel preached, do not follow it. My hope and prayer is that everyone will turn and follow the Lord Jesus Christ. He loves us all. He accepts us all. He takes us from the point of being lost and takes us to a new place of maturity as we grow. We come to Him just as we are and He accepts us exactly as we are, but He doesn't leave us that way. He changes us. But He does it, not us. We don't do it in our own power. That's all I have to say. I kind of got preachy. Sorry. We're in this beautiful place and I got contemplative.

Sheila: Why are you sorry?

Brian: I'm not sorry. The Gospel of Jesus Christ does not change. We don't try to make it "relevant" for today. It's just the way it is. It should bring us to our knees in repentance.

July 13, 2015

We received this devotional from a friend a few days ago. It was a real blessing to us!

9 July 2015

From an article called, "Limping Leaders" Charisma magazine:

Years ago I heard an older pastor talk about Jacob—the proud, defiant, and successful young man in Genesis who wrestled with God and walked with a limp for the remainder of his life. The pastor's point was simple. The best, most trustworthy, and godly leaders walk with a limp. They have been humbled by God and by life, and they've learned to lead out of Christ's strength rather than their own.

Moses fits this model. By the time the Lord called Moses to lead the Hebrews out of Egypt, he was already an old man who had made many mistakes and had been humbled by the realities of life. His resume included being a fugitive guilty of murder, a refugee without a land or people to call his own, and a shepherd in one of the most desolate regions on earth. Not exactly the profile of a powerful leader, but he fit God's purposes nicely. Moses, metaphorically, walked with a limp. He had learned humility and not to trust in his own strength or wisdom.

Young people in the church today hear many messages about pursuing their passion, being an agent of change, or doing something radical. They are often told to stand up and take charge, but who is calling them to sit down and take stock? Our culture celebrates youth and vigor far

more than humility and wisdom. That is why so many of the messages we hear from church leaders are about sprinting, but what we desperately need are spiritually mature voices, like the pastor I heard years ago, emphasizing the virtues of limping.
   Exodus 2:11–15
   Genesis 32:22–28
   1 Timothy 3:1–6

BRIAN ... Reflections on one year. Recorded in Spring 2017
We went to Lexington, Virginia, for the one year stroke anniversary. We called it the one year praise anniversary! Lexington is a charming little town in the heart of the Shenandoah Valley, Virginia. Beautiful area, gorgeous drives. We were reminded of how strikingly beautiful the Valley is and how little we had explored it in our years there.

As we were looking back on a year—and I can see clearly since Sheila has documented this entire process—I was able to see how far God had brought me in a year's time. But yet how far I still needed to go.

I'm reminded of our walk with God. There are times when God affords us the opportunity to look back to see where He has brought us from. Those are times we thank Him for what He's done, how He has been gracious and merciful to bring us so far from where we'd been. But also, the Holy Spirit reminds us of how far we still need to go in this transformation process. He convicts us of things still in our lives that we'd like to get over, get through, in order to get closer to God.

It's kind of coincidental that Sheila just read that piece about Jacob wrestling with the angel. Almost three years out from the stroke at this writing, I was recently sitting at the table the other morning after reading through that story again. We were talking about it. I'm reminded of Jacob's tenacity, his willingness to cling to God no matter what the cost to Him ... because He knows that what God has to offer is what matters. That's my interpretation anyway. God touched his hip, and he walked with a limp the rest of his life. The limp was to remind Jacob of what he had been through, the ordeal of wrestling with the angel.

Yes, I've heard several times from the Lord and received reaffirming words from others as well. I do believe I will be, for the most part, 100 percent healed. But I wouldn't be surprised if God leaves me with a little limp or some little thing to remind me. Maybe nobody else would ever notice it, but I'll know it's there. And that will be to remind me of what God has done, what I've been through—and to not go back to how I was before. We can look back and see where God has brought us and be thankful, but we can't look back and be nostalgic, thinking, "Oh I'd like to go back there because it was so much fun back there." Well, it was and it wasn't.

Sheila: That's a hard thing.

Brian: Yes. It's a hard thing. God's brought you through so much, you've learned new lessons that you can't really go back.

As we were looking at the one year anniversary, that's what I was thinking. I was seeing what Sheila has had to deal with, and I was starting to feel a little better, a little more human. Sheila really has had a load on her shoulders, and she handled it with so much grace and mercy.

We just laid in bed the morning of July 11, 2015 remembering vividly the year before. We just held each other, enjoying the peace and quiet. That was enough. So thankful that we still had each other. I don't know what I would do if I had to go through what she went through! I can't imagine watching all that happen to her, to see her in the condition I was in. That would just tear me up inside. I'm sure it was tearing her up because her world was upside down. So was mine…. Here I am, I lived through it—sort of. I'm not the same. All kinds of emotional issues go through your head— "What if this is as good as it gets? What if I'm like this for the rest of my life?" But then you just have to come back and focus on Christ, realize that it is whatever He wants it to be. And whatever He wants it to be will be fine. You'll get through it. He will be there for you. If He brought you to something, He'll bring you through it!

MORE HOSPITALS

July 15, 2015
Colton driving me to a hospital in mid July. Strange echoes. Garrett is in WMC with possible pneumonia—turned out to be pleurisy in his left lung. Thanks for the prayers.

July 15–17, 2015 Garrett was in Winchester Medical Center with pleurisy. Mac (a homeless man we met at church) was staying with us, which was a blessing because he could stay with Zeppelin. He also cooked for us after we'd spent the night in the ER. The Lord provided a wonderful night nurse who is a devout believer and has a heart for special needs kids. Once I knew Garrett was out of danger, it actually was quite relaxing sleeping and sitting all day in the hospital, resting in quiet... well as quiet as a hospital can be.

July 16, 2015
Hospitals are great for morning people (which I am not). By 6:30 AM all the lights were on and we were off and running ... but here's a verse from my reading today.

Isaiah 50:4 NIV: *"The Sovereign Lord has given me a well-instructed tongue, to know the word that sustains the weary. He wakens me morning by morning, wakens my ear to listen like one being instructed."*

I like the thought of God waking me!

Garrett has been sleeping peacefully all morning. The doctor wants to get him up and moving later to see if his oxygen levels remain good. If they come down with exercise, then she'll likely keep him one more night for observation. Left lung is much better but there is still rattling. However X-rays and CTs are clear. Doctor says "pleurisy"… he's getting strong IV antibiotics, breathing treatments, and good sleep.

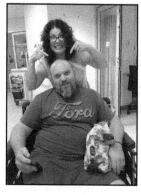

Because we Lloyds like to multitask and use our time wisely:

Brian got here around noon… and guess what? He tripped on the way in to the hospital! He heard a pop and had pain… so we came to the ER to get it checked. Same ER as night of stroke. That's really weird. X-ray was fine… doctor calling it foot sprain. Really?! Ice, feet up, rest… back to doing back flips soon!

July 18, 2015

More multitasking… while Garrett was in the hospital Thursday, we had a new tub/shower put in at home. (The old one was cracked and leaking into the basement! We discovered that last Sunday when we got home from our little Praise Anniversary trip.) Yippee! Then since that is our only bathroom, we have had to farm out showers this week. Brian in all his spare time recovering from the foot injury has finished up the drywall trim and I'll paint… yeah, in the middle of that this afternoon someone wanted to come look at our house who saw it on Craigslist. Okay, Lord! Looking forward to a quiet night! … and hopefully a shower in my own house, lol.

HOUSE FOR SALE

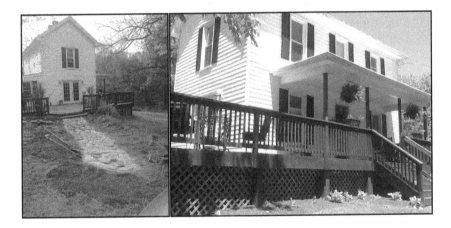

Attention musicians, car enthusiasts, self-employed, work from home....

Charming farmhouse, completely remodeled, on 1 acre in quiet neighborhood, dead-end street. Lovely views, private feel but convenient to towns of Edinburg or Mount Jackson, Virginia, in the heart of the Shenandoah Valley. Easy 81 access. Huge deck and beautiful yard, campfire pit, great outdoor living space. Three-bay detached garage/workshop and finished 400-plus square foot studio with heat and AC. Additional outbuilding wired with electric and audio; could be recording studio or home office. Bought it to stay forever but God is calling us to Texas!

July 19, 2015 Sunday morning

I asked permission of the Father to stay home this morning and soak in some quiet and solitude. Plus Garrett still needs rest. Praise you, Lord, for the time of personal worship and renewal, a new song written, and a chance to journal. Quiet is a balm to my soul. For years I was spoiled and had so much of silence and solitude. Very little of either of those this last year! God is teaching me to find peace in the midst of busyness, chaos, people around, noise. Jesus is my peace.

We attended the wedding of some young friends this afternoon. The long, beautiful drive through lush countryside afforded time for some heart-to-heart conversation about a touchy subject—sex and intimacy in this new season of recovery. We are very grateful for the foundation of years of healthy communication!

During this season, the Lord is transforming my willingness to travel internationally—not just for pleasure or my own agenda—but a true willingness to go wherever **He** calls me to go, for His purposes. It has been a significant dying to self and changing of long-held viewpoints on missionary service as well. I realized that my heart was warming to the idea. That was a surprise to me, and I had to consciously allow it. Growing up, I constantly heard conversations about travel to Africa (present and past) with the challenges as well as the miracles. (There are three generations of missionaries to Chad, Africa, on my mother's side. Beginning in the 1920s with my grandparents.) I never wanted to go. I closed myself off to it at a very young age—I think out of fear… fear of the snakes, the weird food, accommodations, difficult travel schedule. I'm embarrassed to admit that now, but it's the truth. I was the good little Baptist girl who accepted Jesus at five years old and sat in services listening to missionaries say things like, "I know someone here is being called to become a missionary! Are you willing to go wherever God wants you to go and do whatever He wants you to do?" Truly loving God and wanting to be obedient, I would shakily raise my hand and say in my heart, "Yes, Lord. But **please** don't make me go to Africa!!"

*** *Staying home from church that day, the Lord and I had a special time of worship together. It was a Sunday morning but I sensed His permission to bypass normal responsibilities and routines and have some physical rest, solitude, and intimacy with him (all of which I desperately needed as it had been a whirlwind season with lots of demands on me physically, emotionally, and spiritually). During this time, He gave me a new song and part of it was my asking Him to "give me the nations—to put them in my heart." I have no idea what might come from that prayer. But He knows! Ha! So when/if GOD wants me (us) to go, God will supply! His bank account is never at risk as He owns the cattle on a thousand hills.*

Footnote 7/19/17 The Lord so far has not called us to travel to Africa or anywhere else internationally, but we remain open to His plan.

July 21, 2015

We have the house for sale on Craigslist and have had several parties look at it. One couple in particular seem extremely interested, said they are trying to get an appointment at their bank. We will see. When God sells the house we will move.

The Lord continues to reveal things to us—blessings, challenges, things He wants adjusted. Pray for Brian to clearly discern some lessons he is sensing right now.

Although we are excited and anxious to start the new adventure, we trust the Lord's perfect timing.

We are waiting to hear back from Social Services' attorney regarding Garrett's guardianship. We are also waiting for the neurologist about Brian's possibly receiving Botox therapy. (We did not feel a peace about that and in the end it did not come about.) We are praying in the meantime to be used of the Lord however He sees fit here. We sense our calling and passion lifting from the church plant, and that is an odd feeling. Pray that we finish strong for Christ's glory! As a missionary friend says, "God gives you grace to come to an area, and God gives you grace to leave." Very interesting to feel that.

I have officially notified my students; however, I told them I would be teaching lessons as usual until we have a definite date to move.

July 25, 2015 A word in the night: *"He rewards those who earnestly seek him,"* which is taken from Hebrews 11: 6b NIV. The Lord is rewarding us since we are earnestly seeking him.

I was contemplating this whole leap of faith Brian and I are embarking on. Brian's comment: "I guess the worst-case scenario is if we get to Fort Davis, Texas, and we hadn't heard God, he has us live in our truck." But that is not consistent with His character! As a loving Father whose children are honestly trying to seek him, He will bless us! If we don't hear Him completely clearly, He knows our heart and will guide us.

Also a reminder of something from ladies Bible study—Priscilla Shirer's book, Discerning the Voice of God: How to recognize when God is Speaking poses these challenging questions: "What is my motive for pressing in, for seeking the Lord? Do I want to just get direction for my life? To know what to do? Or do I press into the Lord because I want to know God?!"

Forgive me, Lord, and give me a heart to press into you just because I love you and want to know you more.

July 26, 2015

Well, we did get an offer on the house yesterday! I put the house on Facebook Thursday evening and got a lot of comments and stirring over it. Boy, if we wanted to do rent-to-own, we would have had tons of takers! By Friday I had two appointments for Saturday morning.

The second woman who came had done her homework with her bank before she even came to look. She's been looking for a year and knows what she wants. She doesn't need to sell her home before buying ours, so can proceed very quickly. She was building into her offer the consideration that she would add on a master bedroom suite here with a jacuzzi tub. We will see if it all goes through. She works from home (so the studio was appealing). Her boyfriend was with her—very nice people, calm and straightforward.

We also talked with her about the Lord because she opened up and shared how she lost her son nine years ago in a car accident. He was twenty. Wow. I gave her my Healing River CD, which she seemed to really appreciate. They were here over 2 hours. She loves flowers and was excited about the yard.

She was nervous to throw out an offer but Brian encouraged her, said we wouldn't be offended. We haggled a bit back and forth but agreed to a price which would give us a nice profit. We are sort of in shock but are prayerfully trusting....

July 27, 2015

A friend this morning asked for prayer to move in God's rhythm. I love that—move in His rhythm! We are on the way to UVA for checkup. Brian noticed **huge** benefit from chiropractic appointment last Friday. Has another tomorrow.

Consult with sinus surgeon at UVA who did his surgery in January. There is **still** inflammation! Hindsight being 20/20, he wishes he had done the left side at the same time. We'll be back in a month for CT and to determine... good news is that he has a colleague in San Antonio, Texas, whom he trained; he can refer Brian to for follow up. God has it all worked out.

BRIAN: ON SALE OF HOUSE

Monday morning July 27, 2015. We were driving to UVA for a sinus checkup. It was less than 48 hours after we had received a cash offer for our house in Edinburg, VA. That day was, I have to be honest, an "Oh crap!" moment for me. We'd had a lot of big talk about moving, but suddenly things were happening quickly! We'd had the house on Craigslist for a few weeks and received more interest than I had expected. People—a young couple in particular—were pretty serious, but they still had to go to the bank, get things in order.

We came to the point I told Sheila, "We either need to poop or get off the pot. If we're serious about selling this house, let's put it in the hands of a realtor." Now, that, in our area, usually meant a six-month to one-year process at least. Houses weren't moving very quickly at that time. Sheila said, "Before I do that, I'd like to put it on Facebook." I figured, "Okay, fine, what's it going to hurt?" Right. That was a Thursday night. By Saturday afternoon we have an offer. An offer that doesn't require her selling her other house. She just was ready to buy, had been looking for over a year. She had a cabin up in the mountains, but she didn't have to sell it to buy our house.

Sheila: Well, remember we just kept saying, "When God sells the house, we'll move to Fort Davis, Texas." People would ask us, "When are you moving?" Our answer, "When God sells the house."

Brian: I remember thinking, "Okay. She made us an offer. We haggled back and forth a few times and agreed on a price. But, you know, it'll still take a while if we ever do hear back from her." We put it on Facebook Thursday evening. She looked at it Saturday afternoon and made us an offer. I was shocked when she called us at 9:30 AM on our way to the sinus doctor less than 48 hours later! That means either before or between Saturday afternoon and Monday morning at 9:30 AM, she had spoken to the bank, the attorney, and the home inspector. She could close in two weeks! She already had all this done. That is an "Oh crap!" moment. I thought I would have more time to prepare.

There again, that reinforces the idea that God's timing is not our timing. God doesn't always move fast. But when He does move, it's *suddenly.* You know, we'd been building this moment up for two years, and all of a sudden it's here. We've got nineteen years in the Valley that we need to get straightened up in two months. (We put her off and set closing September 30, 2015.) That's the moment, I have to be honest....

Sheila: Me too!

Brian: I thought, "Oh, shoot! We're doing this." I admit there was a lot of mixed emotions in me. I thought, "Are we doing the right thing? Are we really going to do this? Lord, what in the world am I thinking? It's everything I can do to walk on my own without a cane and a walker to get around unassisted. I really can't get around that well right now. I can't get around very quickly, and I have to be very deliberate in how I step because I can lose my balance in a second. How in the world am I going to pack a house, drive across the country, take care of anything that comes up—because Colton is staying in Virginia? Lord, am I insane?!"

God just kind of responded to me in that moment and said, "That's what I want. I want somebody who is insane for Me, who is willing to do stuff that looks crazy, that looks like it doesn't make it any sense. Because that's when the world sees a difference." The world doesn't make any sense. God does, but it doesn't look smart in the world's eyes.

Sheila: Even a lot of Christians thought we were nuts.

Brian: Oh, yeah! I know a lot of our friends and family looked at us like we were nuts. The only people who I think really understood what God was doing was Rob and Tammy Wescoat because they're pretty out of the box thinkers—and God was taking them on an interesting journey as well at the time. Bryan and Aimee for example, I know they love us and are dear friends, but I know they looked at us like, "You're nuts and making a big mistake."

Also, the closest hospital to Fort Davis is 24 miles away and it only has twenty-four beds total. The major hospitals of Odessa/ Midland or El Paso were 2–3 hours away! How does this make sense for a man recovering from a massive stroke?! Again, friends, family, parents, were very gracious and supportive, but I know the doubts and questions were in the back of their minds.

God has shown us in the almost year-and-a-half being out here how He has been faithful. Even the things that have cropped up and we viewed as an emergency—if you had told me ahead of time I'd have thought, "There's just no way I can deal with that right now!"—but we dealt with it. For example, we had to fix the truck on the way out. There was a leak in the transmission, and the o-ring needed to be replaced.

Sheila: It was like a $7 part.

Brian: It could have been terrible. But it ended up being just a $3 or $7 part that I was able to go across the street to the hardware store and was able to fix it right there in the hotel parking lot in Texarkana! I had to prop myself up against the truck in order to do it. Right beside a trailer full of new Corvettes, I remember that, lol. I was hoping no Chevy cooties would get on me.

In this whole adventure, over the course of about a year and two months, we thought about selling, sensed God asking us if we'd be willing to move, then pretty sure God was still going to move us to Texas…to "Oh shoot! We're moving! You're really doing this, God. I was really hoping You were bluffing."

Honestly, there was part of me that was hoping that God was bluffing—we'd have the house for sale for years, and we'd be able to use that as an excuse: "Well, God didn't sell the house." Believe me, I put fleeces up before the Lord, a couple of them, because this move was such a big deal. I made that very private between me and the Lord. Nobody else knew, not even Sheila. I wanted to know for sure. I was not certain; it was such a big step for me.

It would have been one thing if I was perfectly fine physically. I would have been able to say, "Well, sure, I can do this."

Sheila: It still would have been a huge step.

Brian: Yes, but I would have felt like I could do it. That's not what He wanted. That's not what God wanted. It was God saying, "No. *I* can do this!" Not me. Him.

That's a lesson He has taught me over and over again out here. And I think no matter where He carries me from here, that's a lesson I will take with me: He can do all things. I can do all things through Him who strengthens me when He's calling me to do it. When I'm listening to Him. I don't get to choose what those things are. He chooses and I follow. That's all I have to say about that.

July 30, 2015 PUBLIC JOURNAL
With all the challenges and blessings we have been through this past year, I just want to say that I am more in love with my husband now than ever and and that's interesting because it's on a spiritual level. I so respect the character that he has displayed through this test and recovery.

God is simply amazing and when we choose to follow Him ... wow!

July 30, 2015 PRIVATE JOURNAL
Things are moving **fast** regarding our move to Fort Davis, Texas. There are a hundred thoughts swirling in my brain ... **but** I have thought several times about how our experience right now compares to my maternal grandparents' call to Africa, in the mid 1920s. So I'd like to process that a bit.

They were young students at Bible school when they sensed God calling them (individually) to what was then called French Equatorial Africa or Central African Republic. (According to Encyclopedia Britannica, this consisted of four French territories in central Africa from 1910-1959. Chad - or Tchad- had been attached in 1920.) Wanting to make sure they were both called and not just because they were in love following the other's call, they waited for God's confirmation. Receiving it, they married after school and set out.

I thought about that—they were heading to Africa, a country they had never seen, unsure of resources and financial support, knowing they wouldn't see their families for at least the four-year furlough, and facing the possibility that they might never come home at all. We are hearing a call to somewhere within the United States where there are planes, trains, automobiles, not to mention internet, cell phones, Facebook, Skype, FaceTime, texting among other ways to stay in touch! UPS and Fed Express will ship anything to any location, and Amazon is a virtual mall of America! No comparison.

So first of all, thanks, Lord.

The decision to say **yes** and to move is **not** because we have had a really hard year. It is not because we just want a change of pace and scenery. Now, certainly we are weary from this past year and something **new** sounds very good! However, we have dialogued **a lot** together and individually with the Lord to make sure that our desire to move to Texas was not just based on these human reasons. We made it very clear, "Lord if **You** want us to do this, we will. But if this is us and not You, please close the door!" I told my mom that we put out a fleece a few times, particularly in the case of selling the house. We said over and over, "When God sells the house we'll move. It's in His time." She said, "Well, it looks like that fleece is wet." (Yeah, guess so—six weeks on Craigslist and 48 hours on Facebook before receiving an offer!)

I prayed a prayer of surrender about all this international travel stuff while driving to Pennsylvania July 2 for a weekend with my mom and the Mooney Reunion. That weekend with my mom was one of the most precious in my life. There were a couple main things on the agenda: to help her clean out more of dad's stuff and Kevin's room. But I wanted to have some real heart-to-heart talks with her to see how she really was about this whole "moving to Texas thing."

We talked at length about all kinds of things; I was able to share spiritually in depth about what God has been doing—through Brian's stroke, in ministry, in our lives personally, and all of the confirmations of the calling we have received. She responded as she has from the beginning, "Honey, you have to do what you believe God is calling you to do."

While telling her, "Mom, I'm sure some people think we have lost our minds picking up and moving across the country like this. It doesn't make sense to many people—even believers. People just don't operate like this." (Not that we care what people think because that's really **not** what matters!) She said, "Well, that's how my family always operated— if God said, 'Go!' then we went. She said, "Read your grandparents' diaries of those years of early missions in Chad, Africa. They were **full** of descriptions like, 'Today was simply delightful! God is just doing marvelous things! Everything is great!' and so on. But, Sheila, they were living in mud huts with thatched roofs! They had a vehicle which hardly could make it from one town to the other on terrible roads! There were snakes and all kinds of challenges. **But** they were doing what God had called them to do, and they were delighted about it!"

That **so** blessed me! And as I reflected on it later, I realized that what she was also saying was, "Sheila, this is part of your heritage. This is part of your spiritual inheritance—the stepping out into the unknown, pioneering a path led by the Holy Spirit, trusting God to provide and seeing Him work in amazing ways!" Gram's life verse was Isaiah 41:10 and 13 KJV, and on everything she signed her name to she would write, *"I will help thee."*

I never really had felt a connection with the missionary calling until 2013 when God began stirring Fort Davis, Texas, and Sunspot, New Mexico, in our hearts. How can one feel drawn to a place one has never been? And then after a visit of five days, how can one feel homesick for that place? Only through the Spirit of the Living God.

Definitely it is a very interesting time in our lives! We have a contract on the house, and the closing is set for September 30. The administrative tasks loom high, and our minds are filled with questions...**but** we both have peace as the arbiter of our hearts and decisions (Colossians 3:15).

We have sought the Lord the best we know how. We have surrendered and prayed and surrendered some more. We have watched Him do absolute miracles through the past year (from Brian suffering the stroke), and we now stand on the threshold of a new adventure, truly a new way of life. It feels like a fresh start and a whole new mindset. It feels like freedom! I am fully expecting God to do some extraordinary things! We are excited to watch how He is going to provide and guide.

We know that God did not cause the stroke. However, He did allow it … partly to stretch us, to deepen our love, appreciation, and commitment in our marriage, to build our faith muscles and to give us a new vision of His plan for our lives. And truly, after trusting God with the challenges of the past year—my husband's life being spared, our mortgage and bills staying current despite little income, hundreds of thousands of dollars of medical bills being wiped out—trusting God with a little thing like a move to a new land seems fairly easy!

There are just so many aspects, examples, and God stories!—Guerrilla Worship, Scriptures repeated over and over (ex. Isaiah 43:18–19). It's not possible to capture them all or to relay them all. I must trust that when the Lord wants us to share them, He will bring them to mind. The crucible of the last year has been extremely intense, but there has been much refining and much elimination of dross I pray. May we come out like gold to the glory of Jesus' name!

House Sold!

August 7, 2015 PUBLIC JOURNAL

We kept saying, "We will move to Texas when God sells the house."…
Well, He sure moved fast! It was on Facebook less than 48 hours and
we had an offer. Papers were signed yesterday, and closing date is
September 30!

The five years that we have lived in this home have been characterized by peace, rest, healing, hearing God speak, creativity, worship, and
a sense of preparation.

We have loved living here! And yet we are ready to go, and we
are excited about the new adventure to come! The scenery sure will be
different! Still beautiful—simply a different kind of beauty. Still mountains—they just look different because they're not all covered with trees.

We are expecting the Lord to move in mighty ways in Fort Davis,
Texas—perhaps beginning with a new place to live. We can't wait to see
what He does!

BRIAN: FALL MOVING…2015

We're moving! We have all this preparation for moving: finding a
truck, packing up everything, organizing the whole procedure. I had
to rely on friends and family to pack up. I had…how many cars?

Sheila: Oh, my gosh! Well, a three-bay garage.

Brian: Yes. A three-bay garage full of cars and parts.

Sheila: Stuff outside. Stuff at your dad's garage.

Brian. No way I could pack it or move it to where it needed to go. God bless my dad and my son Colton because they worked their butts off getting rid of stuff, taking things down to his garage. Dad's garage was just full! He had my Thunderbird, Colton's truck. Plus, Colton was moving in to their house when we left; so he had his Mustang he was driving and his four-wheel drive truck. It was just a packed house down at Dad's. I know what they put up with, and I appreciate them for doing so.

Sheila: We had all Colton's things to handle separately from all of our belongings. Most of our household was being put in two different storage units in Virginia. Our vehicle was going to be packed up with some essentials and some clothing for the initial journey. We would be heading out October 1 ... not sure where we would live except that we knew we could stay as long as we needed to at our friend Paula's house. Then we weren't sure when we'd be coming back to Virginia to get the rest of our stuff out of storage. It was purely a journey of faith—dependent on how God moved—literally.

Brian: We had so many friends help do things, helping Sheila clean the house, pack the dishes, all the kitchen materials, moving mattresses, getting rid of furniture. A lot of belongings we just got rid of.

I remember the day we were getting ready to leave, putting most things in storage as Sheila mentioned. All we were going to take is what we could fit in Sheila's Mustang that would be hauled on the car trailer, and then in the back of the Expedition. That's what we did on that initial move October 1.

We really didn't have anything planned at first. We truly just winged this whole thing. The whole, "Abraham, go!" thing. Yep. We ended up coming back at Christmastime to empty out the storage units. It really was truly bizarre.

Sheila: I even look back on it now and think, "Wow."

Brian: I guess there are some people who live their lives like this. I am now starting to be able to appreciate it, realizing—hold on to stuff very loosely. It's not about possessions. I don't know how many items we ended up giving away because we didn't want to move it. We thought, "This isn't worth moving across country. We just don't care that much anymore." I know we were able to bless a family with our king-size mattress and some couches. I remember they were so grateful. The husband was going through a hard time physically; he'd had a surgery done and was barely getting back to work. They desperately needed a bed, and we felt we were supposed to just let it go. Even in our hardship—we didn't have a lot of cash—it's not like we were going to go to Fort Davis and buy all new furniture. We didn't have that kind of money! But we just felt God say, "Let it go and let Me provide."

Sheila: And boy, did He ever!

Brian: He provided in such a way that He gave us a house to live in that was physically much bigger than the house we left, had a one-and-a-half car garage for me to play around in, fenced yard, and doggie door for our dog. And the house was totally furnished! We just moved in! I can't begin to understand how God worked....

Sheila: But I think that's the next book.

Brian: Yes, maybe so. But I can't begin to explain the ways God provides if you let Him. Just let go of it. I wish I could put it in better terms to explain it, but I'm simply not able to fully describe it....The peace that comes from knowing Christ. The peace, contentment, and the realization: all the things I chased after for years—there was nothing evil about it—but they were pursuits of the world. Trivial things that do not matter in the grand scheme of things. I'm not going to get to Heaven and have God say, "You know that '65 Ferrari 275 GTB you restored? That was cool! That was the pinnacle of your life." No! He's not going to look at me and say, "Remember that '64 Thunderbird you had? That was boss. That was a bad car." No. He's not going to care about that stuff. He's going to look at me and say, "Remember the time you let the homeless man stay at your house? That blessed me." It's those kinds of things He cares about.

I wasn't even thinking about God's perspective for so long in my life. I was just thinking about me, what I wanted, what could help my career, what could help me advance, what could make our life better. I was worried about the wrong priorities. I had made other things my god. The Lord was starting to show me and purify all of that for the next year-and-a-half in Fort Davis, Texas—that's what that time was about. That might be another story for another time, but it's about Him unraveling all the things I had wrapped my life around—or wrapped around my life. He's still slowly revealing them. Getting me down to the core of who I am in Him—the basic simple truth that He is my Savior and my God. And that's all I really need to know!

August 8, 2015

Word from the Lord through Bryan Patrick: what we have joked about with the "stripping down to the 300" God takes very seriously. We are being stripped down! In our testimony we will see and others will see God's power displayed. Regarding the suffering and the challenges, the Lord does use it for his purposes in our lives.

*** *I did not have a full understanding of this word from the Lord until we had been in Texas a few months. Actually, the implications of being "stripped down" continued throughout our time there. We were stripped down in every way! And the Lord had lessons to teach us. I spent much time and many journal pages processing it all and capturing the insights the Lord was giving through it all. He removed every "prop" we had in order to whittle both of us down to our core identity in Him ... and then He built us back up as only He can do. The physical "stripping" with the stroke for Brian is pretty obvious, but there were so many deeper, invisible, emotional/relational/spiritual issues in each of us addressed as well. Our time in the desert is quite fascinating ... and ultimately, by God's grace, rejuvenating. But again, that is a topic for the next book if God allows.*

August 17, 2015

Psalm 36:8 NIV
"They feast on the abundance of your house; you give them drink from your river of delights."

I want to drink from **that** river! And we have an open invitation!

August 18, 2015
PRAISE REPORT...

A few weeks ago we finally were allowed to fill out financial aid paperwork regarding the PHII medical helicopter bill. Anthem had paid 7,000 of the $41,000 bill. Aimee Patrick had been speaking with one representative for months and months. She called again and got someone else who gave some great advice. We sent in financial aid paperwork along with a detailed letter a few weeks ago. **Today** Aimee called and was told they are still reviewing it with the committee, but everything looks very good. Sounds like it's all going to be taken care of! God is amazing! Thank you, Lord!

August 19, 2015

Sometimes God's chosen response is silence. Hmmmm. True. Psalm 46:10. So, will I choose to just continue to trust in Him and fall on Him?

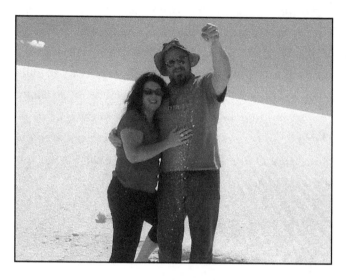

August 20, 2015 Blessing and Bon Voyage

Please share and consider yourself invited! Party September 20 at Woodstock Park, 3:00-6:00PM

Photo is from our visit to White Sands, New Mexico, in August 2013

SECOND SINUS SURGERY?!

August 25, 2015

Today once again we travel to UVA to meet with a sinus surgeon. He will determine if Brian needs to have surgery on the left side of his sinuses. Appreciate prayers. We're fine if that needs to happen.... At this point we just want it done and him healed!

Well... we are sitting in a **packed** waiting room at UVA for pre-op for sinus surgery. We're on standby for the surgery date—hopefully September 10.

August 26, 2015

Yesterday was a long day! By the time we had CT, appointment with doctor, preregistered at UVA and then picked up G, we didn't get home until after 4:00 PM. But we enjoyed the time together and the beautiful drive. We had great conversations.

Yes, we are off to the races with another sinus surgery! There are definitely issues on the left side of his sinuses, as well as a couple things still on the right side need to be corrected. They are simple things, but they need to be done.

We are on standby for time in the operating room, hopefully the morning of September 10. That's great because you know we have nothing else going on in September! Lol, but truly we are hoping it works because we would like this doctor to do it.

We are both fine and at peace with the decision. God's got it! Thank you for your concern and prayers!

August 25, 2015
Brian: Second sinus surgery?!

This is God's sense of humor and the way God works: in a little over a year's time I've had a stroke, two sinus surgeries, and we're moving across the country to Southwest Texas! What in the world?! You know, if we were to look at our life from the outside looking in, we would think, "These people are going to explode!"

I can't begin to describe to you the way God worked it out. I think it's because He just wanted it all done and out of the way. Maybe He said, "It's going to be a hellish year. Throw this year away. But we're going to get all of this mess out of the way instead of drawing it out over the course of the next ten years."

*Sheila: Yes, but also I think He wanted there to be **no** doubt—to us or to anybody else watching—that it's **only** His strength. It's only by His strength!*

Brian: Right.

*Sheila: Remember that old study by Henry Blackaby, Experiencing God? That was the first group study we did when we moved to Virginia in 1996. One of the main points was, "If you're feeling like God is calling you to do something and you feel like you can do it, then it's probably not God. On the other hand, if you feel like God is calling you to do something and you feel like there's no way you **can** do it, then you know that it's something **only** God can do!" (See www.lifeway.com for purchase info.)*

Brian: If I'd have looked at anybody else's life going through this, I'd have thought that just the stroke would have been enough! I'd have thought, "Dear God, you had a stroke. You took that year and really recovered. God bless you because that's a stressful year!"

But with us—the stroke, two sinus surgeries, and selling house to move across the country to a town where we really only knew a handful of people—we moved away from our entire support system and away from some of the best hospitals and doctors in the country (INOVA in Fairfax, VA and UVA in Charlottesville, VA). The closest hospital to us in Fort Davis is 24 miles away, and it has twenty-four beds total. So if it's anything really serious, that's just a place where you wait for the helicopter to fly you to Odessa or Dallas or El Paso! It's bizarre.

God wanted to show us that **He** is our support system no matter where we are.

It's funny looking back at this we can really laugh, thank God, and say, "Only God!" But truthfully, **ONLY God**! Only God could have sustained me through this. Through all of this process at that time (Fall 2015) I'd get tired if I had to do too much of anything. I'd get mentally tired. And He allowed me to load a car on a trailer, drive that truck and trailer the whole 1,800 miles across country!

Sheila: Oh that's right, because I didn't drive it with the trailer.

Brian: No. I didn't want you driving the trailer because you weren't used to that. I drove that truck the entire way, and I was good! God blessed me with strength and perseverance so that I was fine. I was able to get out and fix it when that o-ring started leaking transmission fluid; it didn't burn up the transmission or anything. I was able to get to a store, get the part and fix it myself, and get back on the road the next day. We didn't even lose a lot of time. I can't begin to tell you what a miracle that is in and of itself! You don't realize it at the time. When I look back on it I think, "How in the world was I able to do that?!" Even today (April 2017) if I think about getting in the truck and hauling a trailer all the way across country as the only driver, I'd say, "I'm nuts! There's no way I can do that right now." But I did it a year-and-a-half ago!

Sheila: Because God wanted you to.

Brian: So don't ever doubt that God can do something. And that's just a small example compared to what some people have gone through in their lives. I realize that. I'm not trying to make myself out to be some kind of major martyr for Christ. I went through some physical issues. Due to the grace of God I'm still here, able to write this down. (Or speak it, actually. I'm not writing anything, talking into Sheila's iPhone.)

He showed me in this process that He is my Strength, He is my Provider, He is my Comforter in everything! But I have to let go of my life.

It's an odd feeling when you're packing up and driving away from the house you've known and loved...we honestly thought when we bought that house that we could retire there, live the rest of our lives right there. We loved that place. However, God called us.

I ask you once again: what are you willing to give up to follow Jesus? And the answer is *everything*. The answer is always everything. What aren't you willing to give up? If there's something you aren't willing to give up to follow Christ, you need to really think about your relationship with that thing. There should be nothing between you and God. There should be nothing that you cling to so tightly that you can't let go to follow the Lord.

MOVING PREPARATIONS

August 26, 2015
Zep guarding the boxes?! We are hoping to get the storage unit today. Then we will be asking for help! The plan is to put everything in storage here, stay with friends in Fort Davis until we have a sense of where God has for us to live... then we will come back and get it all. Brian is not able to carry stuff, so help is appreciated! Thanks

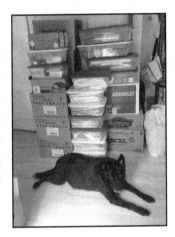

September 10, 2015 PRIVATE EMAIL TO A CLOSE FRIEND

How am I feeling? I'm doing OK.

Reality hit me the other day because I told a couple of my piano students that next week would be their last lesson. That hit me! I love these kids. I enjoy teaching and have taught lessons here in the Valley for nineteen years.

There is such a mixture of emotions. I am really excited and looking forward to the new adventure! We know beyond a doubt that it is what God is calling us to do. However, it feels strange to pick up roots and move in such a big way.

To be honest, I have not been focusing on my feelings that much. Remember that line up prayer? The fact is that I made a decision to obey, and I'm walking that out. (The so-called "line up" prayer is declaring submission to God's order: I am surrendered spirit, body, and soul—including mind, will, and emotions—to the Lord.)

I think this past year has actually been good practice for this change. Our lives were completely turned upside down July 10, 2014. Consequently, it's been an entire year of adjusting and dealing with feelings all over the spectrum.

A mom of a student last night asked me, "How are you handling all of this... teaching, doctor appointments, moving, family?" I replied, "By the grace of God. One day at a time."

That sounds trite, but it's true. The Word promises that for those who love and trust Him, the Lord moves us from strength to strength (Psalm 84); He gives us grace and strength in the moment we need it. I have lived that in a whole new way this last year.

September 12, 2015

Cleaning out the garage today with my men, making a casserole to attend a wedding tonight, church, and then playing music for a church tomorrow afternoon, Brian's sinus surgery Monday. Ugh. Strength, Lord Jesus!

*** *Looking back, at this point, honestly, I was just kind of in a zone. There was **so** much to be done on so many emotional as well as physical levels, that I just kept moving. I kept focusing on the next step right in front of me and plugged along. Sleep was not a commodity in abundance! I'd fall sound asleep but if I woke up, my mind would just start spinning with everything that was happening and that needed to be done. No doubt the Lord gave me strength and kept me healthy. It makes more sense though now why I was utterly exhausted by the time we arrived in Fort Davis less than one month later. You go from 100 mph all the time to nothing on your plate at all except getting Garrett back and forth to school. That began a new season of adjustment and **rest** in the Lord ... but that's a story for another time.*

September 13, 2015

Brian ... sinus surgery round two ... tomorrow. We need to arrive at UVA at 11:30 AM. That's good news/bad news ... we can get G on the bus but Brian has to be fasting!

September 14, 2015

Update on Brian's sinus surgery ...

The doctor just called. He's done. There was quite a bit of oozing blood during surgery, lots of inflammation in there. They did need to straighten out his septum, and the bone was thick. That took a while. Narrow nose passages. But he is fine; the doctor said they accomplished all their goals! Nurse from recovery says he is still asleep but will call me soon to come up. Praise God!

September 14, 2015

Good trip home—thanks for the prayers. Couple stops and got home around 10:15 PM. He spent night on recliner but couldn't sleep at all (steroids in IV?). I slept wonderfully. He feels okay, just would like to sleep! Pray he can. He's allowed to use his CPAP today.

September 16, 2015

My hubby preaches Sunday September 20 at 10:00 AM at Fresh Water Fellowship. All are welcome! Then our bon voyage party is Sunday afternoon 3:00–6:00 PM at Woodstock Park. Please stop in!

September 17, 2015

Brian notices a **huge** improvement this morning (after the second sinus surgery Monday September 14). Feels the infection is gone—physically and spiritually. Feeding the flesh is like infection. He can move his left arm, hand, wrist this morning in ways he couldn't even two days ago. **Praise the Lord**! He can go down steps easily. The swelling in his legs/feet is minimal. He's been peeing a ton (getting rid of infection?). We are trusting this is healing, not just the steroids. The "pressure cap" feeling around his head that has been there since the stroke is gone!

I have a retreat today. He said he's going out to studio to spend time with the Father, pray and try to play guitar.

September 18, 2015

Update on Brian: he is really feeling good! He notices more fluidity in his left side since the sinus surgery on Monday. There is much less swelling in his legs and ankles as well. His voice is stronger because the airflow is unobstructed. Oxygen is an important thing! We are very grateful to God!

*** *Unfortunately when the steroids wore off, much of the stiffness returned, as did the "skull cap." That was really discouraging.*

CREDIT CARDS

September 18, 2015

Well, we have finally received notice from Discover card. They are sending our account to an attorney unless we make arrangements/payment by the end of October. God clearly told Brian in May that He's got it. The card is only in my name, and B has sensed that is significant. Please pray for our discernment in this matter. Above all we want to obey God. And also, according to the Jewish calendar, it's the year of Jubilee … which is interesting to ponder during this time. We will have the money after the close of the house….

BRIAN: CREDIT CARDS

One credit card was taken care of earlier, but I told you the second one was a long drawn-out process. Chase Visa, the first credit card company, worked with us as soon as Sheila called a couple weeks after the stroke. They were fairly accommodating and later settled for pennies on the dollar.

However, Discover credit card company was never willing to work with us, even though Sheila had been a member in good standing since 1986! The couple instances over thirty years she'd been accidentally late on a payment, she would call to let them know. Because my name wasn't on the card, they would only talk to Sheila. Despite her best efforts—and my wife is incredibly per-severant!—they were not willing to take a settlement.

We were proactive very soon after the stroke and in the months to follow, keeping them informed of our situation. For several months we were able to continue making the payments. What I felt when I heard Sheila on the phone with them finally was, "Look, you've done everything. You've been honorable trying to tell them when and why you'd have to start missing payments. You were humble. You didn't make excuses; you just gave the facts." Then I felt the Lord said, "We all owe a debt we cannot pay. You've been more than straight up with these people. Trust me. I'll take care of it. I will pay this debt."

Now, I didn't know what that meant. I didn't know how it was going to play out. We didn't know exactly actually **until** we moved. God had taken care of everything else I had asked about. Remember I mentioned the fleeces I put before the Lord? He had met every one of them except for this last debt. This was one specific thing I had talked to Him about, and I was struggling not having it resolved before we set out on the move. Finally, I sensed He said, "I've taken care of everything else for you. Will you trust me with this? It will be taken care of. This will not leave you in a bind. It will not take that big of a chunk out of the profit you made from the sale of the house. Trust me on this."
So we did, and we moved.

But after we moved—two weeks after we arrived in Fort Davis, Texas—God took care of it. In a mighty way. Now we are completely debt-free! God took us from having a house payment, credit card payments, living paycheck to paycheck—like many typical American households—to having a stroke and no income on my end. (Sheila still had some income from piano lessons, although she had to miss some at times with therapy/doctor appointments, etc.). Way more than half our income had been cut out. And yet God used all of that to get us completely out of debt! It's absolutely amazing how the Lord took care of us financially! It makes no sense in the world system…just God. And we are incredibly grateful.

Sheila: God's math is different.

Brian: We're learning to let God lead, rely on God instead of relying on Brian and Sheila. When you rely on God, He is a much better Provider than you are! And it's not about the money. I'm not saying this is the formula for getting out of debt. This is **not** promoting the "gospel" of prosperity that plagues the Church in our culture. I'm simply saying, "Let God do it. He's better at solving problems than you are anyway!" He knows exactly how everything works. We only have clues. We only think we understand how things work. God knows how to make things work. So why would you not rely on Him to solve the problem?

CLOSURE AND SAYING GOODBYE ...

September 19, 2015

My last piano recital in Virginia with my students. It was a precious time, although bittersweet. The Lord had me write a "blessing, an encouragement" for each student. I gave it to them (parchment paper rolled up and tied with ribbon) after they played. It was a rich day in which the Lord allowed me to see the positive impact I'd had on people's lives. I had the sense that I had used His gifts to good purpose and that I had "finished well." The end of an era.

September 20, 2015

Our church family hosted a "Bon Voyage" party for us at the Woodstock Park. It was lovely! Beautiful weather and many hugs and well wishes from friends over the nineteen years of life in the Valley.

*** *Looking back, I'll say again that there were many instances in which this was such a surreal experience. At times my heart wrenched at the idea of leaving and going so far away. But truly, the majority of this time of preparation we felt such a sense of anticipation and expectation! We knew beyond a doubt that God was calling us and had a larger plan than we could imagine. The Bible promises that His plans are for our* *good and give us hope. (Jeremiah 29:11, my mom's favorite verse) The feeling of knowing you are following God's call to the best of your ability is extremely gratifying. The peace of Christ covered us and allowed us to make this step of faith. Despite the challenges and difficulties, we felt very "alive."*

September 24, 2015

Heading to UVA for checkup with sinus surgeon. He's had a harder time with this recovery. This was more extensive surgery and involved both sides. When steroids wore off Tuesday he was miserable! Better today and praying for good report. Moving process is going well.

September 27, 2015 our last Sunday in Virginia

Such a special weekend packed with friends, worship, reflection, laughter and tears. **Thank you,** family of Fresh Water Fellowship and dear friend, Pastor Bryan Patrick, for all of your kind words, love and prayers this morning. We felt incredibly honored and supported—what a great "send off" into the next assignment the Lord has for us. We love you all!

I was at the retreat from Friday afternoon 'til Saturday evening. Was **so precious!** Much of it was spent in silence, and what the Lord gave me during that time was a real blessing. Weird to return home to the house being nearly empty.

Here's my Facebook post this morning:

As all the furniture was cleared out of our home yesterday—a **big** thank you to everyone who helped—I was leading worship at a retreat that I'd committed to a few months ago. I questioned the timing as it grew closer, but I knew God wanted me to go. It was held at a gorgeous facility called Mountain Valley Retreat Center, part of Camp Horizons. John and Kim Delaney Kirkpatrick made the trip down from Pennsylvania. Kim, a friend since childhood, came to the retreat with me; John helped the men move.

At a retreat whose theme was *"got prayer?"* twenty-four ladies were asked to fast from words for a period of several hours—a small miracle in itself! Obviously we were encouraged to talk to God, just not one another. We were given scripture to meditate on, including Ephesians 3:16 NIV, *"I pray that out of his glorious riches he may strengthen you with power through his Spirit in your inner being...."*

I fell asleep meditating on that Scripture, listening to light rain on a metal roof in a charming farmhouse surrounded by the gorgeous Virginia Blue Ridge Mountains. I have not slept that soundly in a long time. It was a precious time with the Lord! And one that I would not have experienced if I had not been silent.

I realized later, that was a fitting way to spend my last weekend in Virginia, since leading retreats has been a large part of my ministry in Virginia for years!

Thank you, Lord, for setting aside that time for me way before I knew that it would be my last weekend.

Mixed emotions today as it is our last official Sunday at Fresh Water ... but once again ... excited for the new journey. Feeling like Abraham in Genesis 12.

From friend and prayer partner Vicki N September 27, 2015

As I was reflecting on your FB post and praying over it, I got such a clear sense that the rain that fell through the night was representative of God's peace, mercy, grace, and pleasure with the trust you have in Him and your obedience to Him. It was more than words can express, an anointing of all that is to come.

September 28, 2015 PUBLIC JOURNAL

The kitchen is almost totally cleared out. Have to get the few things left in the bathroom. Cleaning tomorrow ... Brian is fixing something on Expedition.... Please keep us in prayer as I know you have been! Home stretch but we are pooped. Lol

September 28, 2015 PRIVATE JOURNAL

What keeps coming to my mind—as we admit that in our flesh there are many ways we do not want to leave—is the verse (about King David in 2 Samuel 24:24 NIV) *"I will not sacrifice to the Lord my God burnt offerings that cost me nothing."*

And both Brian and I have sensed the Lord acknowledging that cost and assuring of His recompense. We love this home, friends, ministry....

Shared this with a friend. Her response: "Yes and our wants plus fifty cents won't expand the reign of Christ in us. There is always a cost. This one seems high now but later...." Amen!

September 30, 2015 Facebook post

Well, we are officially homeless! Closing all done. And it doesn't feel hopeless at all! In fact, just the opposite! Thank you, Lord! Bless the new owners in their new home in Jesus' name.

Last day ... load to storage and the dump ... then pack up vehicles for the trip. Anybody home with a truck? I prayed for it not to rain today, and look at the patch of **blue sky** over my house! Autumn is my favorite time of year, especially here in the Valley. And it has been raining pretty much straight for the last six days due to a hurricane coming up the coast, so I think it's God's way of making it easier for me to leave.

*** *I'm sure one of the main things people realize as they're moving is how much junk we humans collect! This was really a sobering and rather disgusting realization. We had only been in that house five years, so that means we had moved and cleared everything out. But we were doing it again. And even when we got settled in Fort Davis, Texas, we still had junk in storage. It's amazing how very little we actually need to survive! We pay to maintain it, then pay to move it and often still pay to store whatever doesn't fit in the house. I pray I have learned some lessons from this in how to let go.*

Homeless ... But Invigorated!

BRIAN: GOD MADE US TOTALLY FREE TO GO WHEREVER GOD LEADS US

September 30, 2015

Closed on our house. It's gone. It's not ours anymore. It's hers. As much as we loved it and we kind of wept over leaving it, it also felt good to be free. God freed us up.

Now, we had not been in danger of losing the house. The fact is we could have stayed there. Financially we would have been fine to stay there. But we took the step of faith and therefore were now totally free, completely free to go wherever we sensed the Lord calling us. That was an amazing feeling at forty-seven years old!

We were concerned about Garrett (our then eighteen-year-old son with Down's syndrome and Autism) because he goes with us, and we want to know that he is taken care of. However, we knew he would be taken care of because of...God. I know Sheila had mixed emotions, and I did too. However, we were able to look at each other in the eye after we sold it—maybe with a little tear because we did like it— and realize this is what freedom feels like! We're free! We're free!

That is what God does when you receive Jesus as Savior too! You're free! You're free to follow Him, free to let go of sin…the sin that you think you like, the world that you think you can't live without…you think you're happy. You don't realize how much of a slave you are to it until you let go. You're free!

And we are free. God has freed us of the burden of stuff. When you have stuff, you have to take care of it. You have to maintain it. It's a burden. I'm not saying the Lord will never call us back into having our own place. I'm not saying that. But I'm saying we had to realize how much freer we felt without anything, being essentially homeless!

When we got in the truck to leave October 1, 2015—the next day— it was truly amazing. We just felt like we were embarking on a journey, an adventure. We thought, "Well, Lord, okay. Let's see where You're going to lead." We really were. I never thought it would feel that way. Leading up to it, I never thought about how the freedom would feel.

I prayed for extra angels to watch over that old Expedition with 200,000 miles on it. His angels are better mechanics than I am! They kept that thing running perfectly, except for that little $7 o-ring. Yep. And even that wasn't deadly. We could have kept a watch on the fluid, but it was making a mess. But He allowed me to fix it and fix it cheaply. It was such a sigh of relief.

Moving out we just felt like, "We could stop anywhere!" If God tells us, "You know what? You're not going to Texas. You're going to Montana or Utah or Arkansas or Tennessee. Just stay here; you don't have to go the whole way out." We could say, "Okay!" We had as much chance of a life and a home somewhere else as we did in Fort Davis, Texas! But God worked it out perfectly. Like I said, that's a bigger story—not for this book, maybe another book— I don't know.

You just can't know until you go through it. I believe that's why God is taking us through it. Until you go through the valleys, you don't understand the mountaintops. You don't understand the way God takes care of you through the trials. When we're in the midst of it all, what we can focus on is just putting one foot in front of the other....

Sheila: Just surviving.

Brian: That's all we can really do. We're surviving. But when you're able to look back at the hard times—as we have done in the process of writing this book— you're able to see where God's hand was in **countless** things! We didn't even realize it until after the fact. So just....

Sheila: Trust.

Brian: Trust Him, put one foot in front of the other and say, "Jesus, give me the strength to take another step. And I will take another step. That's all I can do."

When you have those tough times, the bad news, the rough patches, when tragedy happens —and tragedy happens!— trust Him. It doesn't mean the hard times don't hurt. God didn't take away our pain and our struggle. What He did was that He gave me the strength to put one foot in front of the other. Just take that next step. Realize, "Okay, God, I don't know where You're going, but I'm a step closer. I will go wherever You lead me. I can't see the map. All I can see is my foot. One foot in front of the other right now. That's all I can do."

Sheila: And His hand—He lets us see enough to see His hand.

Brian: Well, He lets you feel His hand on you, feel Him. It's a weird thing: people say when a tragic thing first strikes, you think, "My

God, I can't go any farther. I'm done!" There were so many times in this process that I fell to my knees and said, "Okay, I'm done. God, take me. I'd rather be with You and be done with this whole mess than to live like this anymore. I'm tired. I'm frustrated and I want to go home."

But He gives you the resolve. He gives it to you … "Just see if you can stand." If you can stand, He says, "See, you can stand. Now see if you can take a little step." And it's everything you can do to take that next step. "OK, take one more." So you take one more. The weird thing is I don't care if the situation gets better or not. The steps become easier to take with each one. You find, "Okay, I can do it. I can do it, God. You're there. You're helping me. I can feel you. I can do this next step. Okay, yep, I can do the next one. I can do it. I can do it. I can do it because I trust You."

The steps become easier. Before you know it, the steps are light. It doesn't mean that things don't still hurt and that life isn't a little difficult at times. It doesn't mean that you never question God. He can take the questions. He has the answers. He **is** the answer. The steps become easier and easier.

For anybody reading this or listening to this who is going through something hard, whatever it might be, I can think of so many things people have gone through that are harder than what I've gone through….

But I can tell you this: you'll get through it with Jesus. You will get through it. There is a tomorrow. There is a brighter day coming. We know ultimately we have the promise that is Him. This world is really not our home. We are going to be with Him in perfection one day. That is a promise we have! And once we're there, **all** the cares of this life will be gone! We won't care one iota about what we had to go through to get there. We just won't care. It will seem like nothing. Take hope and have faith.

*** *This has been such an interesting journey! Fascinating, grueling, enlightening, growing, refining, agonizing, sad, joyful, inspiring, depressing, and many other adjectives I could use. Obviously if you have read through this book you can clearly see the differences in mine and Brian's personalities as well as perspectives— a fact that has often made life even more colorful. We sincerely hope that by sharing our story you have received encouragement and have drawn closer to the Lord Jesus, who loves you dearly and who is just as involved in your story as He has been in ours.*

Epilogue

April 23, 2017 BRIAN'S REFLECTIONS ON NOW

While talking to a friend of mine, he reminded me of this: he was watching something on the internet about the ministry called Joni's Kids, with Joni Erickson Tada. She's been a quadriplegic for roughly forty years, severely handicapped by a diving accident when she was a teenager. But yet, you look at the way God has used her and worked in her life! She is able to say now that she views her handicap as a blessing because she would not have learned all that she has learned in God if she had been able to continue on the path she'd been on before the accident.

I have to admit that I'm not there. However, I think it's important that we understand how significant the seemingly little things are in the journey.

We look for the big things; we look for the big blessings and sometimes we don't see the little blessings until after the fact. Then we realize, look, God's been there all along, doing this, doing that, working in this way and we didn't even realize it; we weren't even thankful until now.

When you realize those workings of God, as it says in Philippians, we offer our prayers up to God in thankfulness. In gratitude. You're being honest with God about what you need or what you think you need, but you're also thanking Him for what He's done and Who He is. Never forget that.

Sheila: Because also the Scripture says, "Give thanks for all things and in all things." 1 Thes. 5:16-18

Brian: Rejoice in the Lord always and again I say rejoice. And it says if you do these things—I think those verses are in that particular order for a reason, it's Philippians 4:4-9—it says and you will have the peace of God which surpasses all understanding. Because your hope will then truly be in God, not in mankind, not in the world. Hope in the world or in mankind will always fail us, will always let us down because it's not focused on Christ.

What has the Lord taught me through this journey? He has shown me that healing is a lot of times a process that He uses to teach us things. If we shortcut the process, we shortcut ourselves and miss things we need. My physical healing was only the mirror to what God was wanting to do spiritually. He had to strip me down to the minimum, so He could build me back up in him. He peeled me back like an onion a layer at a time, slowly teaching me the simplicity of His saving grace and the freedom that faith in Jesus brings. By letting things go, I've learned that truly Jesus is all I need. All the stuff I thought I needed to make me happy was really keeping me from experiencing the freedom of Christ. I was a slave to my stuff instead of a slave to Jesus. With each layer of the world he removed, He revealed a deeper spiritual reality.

August 2, 2017

Brian, you have stated that you were a big-picture person. I believe the big picture and the bottom line are important, but the process is important too. The details of how you got to the destination—those are necessary too.

Brian: But everybody's process is different. So if I tell you about my process, that's missing the point. It's not like I've arrived. It's the realization that I am arriving as God transforms my life.

Our individualized process is something God teaches each of us—we need to walk with Him long enough to believe that He really loves us and that He is getting each of us where He needs us to be.

If I try to share with you the process God has used to shape my current relationship with Him, what will happen is that someone will hear it and try to recreate it. That's what we do as humans. This is not a learnable program. It's not as though you can be taught **how** to do it. That's not really what you're needing. You're not learning a definable process. You're growing in a relationship with a living God. He will speak to you and teach you what you need to know. That's between you and God!

If I could get across anything to anybody through this book or through talking in person, it's that your life, your theology, your spiritual growth is between you and God. Nobody else can give it to you. But if you're not willing to put in the time to get to know God, you won't get it. You can't do it any other way. You can read my book, say, or you could read so and so's book, *Twelve Steps to a Better Walk with God.* You can read articles by other people and gain insight because they do contain truth if they are submitted to the Lord. But we cannot put the same weight of application on them as we can from the Bible. Even as you're reading this book, our book is not truth. We are pointing to Truth. We're telling you how the truth of God's promises have influenced our lives.

Read **His** book. Simply get alone with God daily and read. Talk to Him. Let Him talk to you. The main way He talks to you is through His Word. But if you don't read the Word, if you're not getting that, then you're not communicating with God. You're not allowing Him to communicate with you. He's not going to hit you over the head and talk to you like Noah. We all look at the Old

Testament and think, "How much easier would it be if the Lord spoke that directly?" He doesn't always do that. We have the Holy Spirit inside us—if we have believed in Jesus Christ as Savior and Lord—and the Lord gave us a book through which He speaks to us. That Spirit uses the Bible to interpret for our lives—our individual lives—how God wants us to learn from Him.

Sheila: Yes.

Brian: That's the greatest thing I could tell you. That is the greatest gift on this earth, the Word of God, the Bible. It teaches us everything we need to know about God. You wouldn't need to read another book in your life; but if you just read the Bible, I guarantee you that you'll learn everything you need to know about your life with God.

Many people look at every other book **but** the Bible because they're intimidated by it, or maybe they feel inferior because they don't understand what He's trying to say. Just read it! Pick it up and read it! Do what I do—yes, I spend some time studying, but I also simply read through it sometimes as a regular book. Just read through it. I guarantee things will be highlighted to you. You'll stop and you'll reread them. Then take those things and pray about them. Let God talk to you about those things. There's no other process than that! And pray about what He shows you. Let Him speak to you. However, you need to be alone and be quiet so you can hear Him.

Sheila: That reminds me of the song I wrote called "Hear Your Heart"... His whisper becomes like a megaphone to our soul.

Brian: You can hear that still small Voice when you're quiet and waiting before God. It is a still small Voice because God wants you to want Him hard enough, badly enough, that you're willing to shut everything off and just hear Him. Satan's voice is really loud, very boisterous, with tons of noise…because there's no substance. God's voice is quiet and still because it's ALL substance.

If we would just learn to listen to God! Listen to Him! He has something He wants to talk to you about desperately. He wants to talk to each one of us. We don't need to get that message from our pastor or a TV evangelist or from the latest book. We can get that message right from the Source! Yes, insights from others can be good and helpful, as they are directed toward the Truth, but that is not where you get your relationship with God. You get it from yourself being intimate with Him, letting Him talk to you through His word. Through prayer. Through the meditation where He just quietly talks to you and helps you interpret what you read and what you were praying about. Don't sell that short!

Sheila: And don't think you can't have it.

Brian: Right. Don't think you can do without it. It's the Living Water. So when you try to do without it, you dry up! We're out here in the desert physically, but spiritually I'm being watered like never before. I didn't realize that although I was in a lush, green beautiful environment before, spiritually I was living in a desert.

SHEILA'S CONCLUSION WRITTEN
SEPTEMBER 2017

What did i learn through the stroke? How I am more like Jesus because of this experience? **I will admit when one of my editors posed these questions to me**, I was at a loss. I had journaled so avidly throughout the ordeal that the idea of going back and processing that question was rather overwhelming to me. I thought, "Can't the reader glean all those insights through my journal entries?" The answer to that inquiry is, "No."

So ... as I am flying in a plane at 20,000-plus feet, I will endeavor to dive into that question and see what happens. Couldn't pay me to strap on a parachute and jump, but then again this kind of feels just as precarious.

Do I wish the stroke had never happened? Yes! And No! What doesn't kill us makes us stronger. And in the timeless words of Winnie the Pooh to his best little pink friend Piglet, "You are stronger than you think." Now, please understand that I am not trying to glorify myself or my own strength! Sheila, in the flesh, had no bucket from which to draw water from the deep well of the life-altering trauma the stroke had brought into our lives. However, as 2 Corinthians 12:9–10 says, "I will boast all the more gladly in my weaknesses so that Christ's power may rest on me ... when I am weak **then** I am strong. God's power is made perfect in weakness."

At this writing, we are three years, two months since the stroke. We have traveled many miles—physically, emotionally, and spiritually to the moon and back. I have railed screaming, fists raised, at the heavens with the gut-wrenching wail, "**Why?!**" I have soaked my old carpet with tears wrought from an internal void I didn't think would ever be filled. I have looked out at the desert climate with eyes glazed over wanting desperately to go back to LBS (an acronym a friend lovingly tagged for "Life Before Stroke.") I have often wondered how we could continue living in this new reality. Why did things have to change so drastically?

And then one day I realized that I was no longer just surviving. We were no longer just recovering, or even the next phase, recuperating. We were starting to live again, to dream, to laugh truly without the empty horror lurking behind the edges. There is Life After Stroke.

There are still times when I wish Brian could be physically the big, bold, strong-as-an-ox football-player build of a man as he was before the stroke. He still experiences deficiencies and weaknesses due to that blasted brain bleed. The Lord has not **yet** fully restored his ability to play guitar or have the lightning-quick reflexes normally contained in a functioning human hand. Does that mean that I didn't hear God about "full, complete restoration, better than new" in those first hours and days? No! One thing I have learned loudly and clearly: God's timing is not my timing. His ways are not my ways. His thoughts are higher than my thoughts. (Isaiah 55:10) I believe now, as I have from the beginning, that the Lord could completely restore Brian in the fraction of a blink. And He is. But it is a process. And if you remember reading early on, Brian surrendered to that process. Numerous times I have had to surrender to the process as well.

The ways in which the Lord **has** restored Brian are amazing; truly at times I shake my head in gratitude. First of all, his cognitive abilities were really not affected; he remains quick-witted, wise, discerning, and a bottom-line assessor. Yet his compassion, patience, perseverance, and empathy for others has grown exponentially. The benefits of this to a wife and two sons sharing his home spread like a wide, warm blanket.

In the time afforded him to reflect on his life and commune with the

Lord, he has acknowledged shortcomings or oversights in our relationship or in his character in general. When he has chosen to share with me or ask forgiveness or even acknowledge my strengths and character, I have experienced a soothing balm to my soul, love and healing on a deep level. I know many women who would give anything for a similar experience.

I have learned that the vows one says at a wedding ceremony can truly be put to the test through a traumatic health event. True love comes only from Jesus but can flow out of us and between us if allowed. Marriage is more than passion, financial agreement, success, or even friendship. It is a commitment. And I've learned that when those stormy seas are navigated (again—only by the grace of God), the ensuing relationship is sweeter, deeper, and stronger for having survived the battle.

I've learned some things about myself, about God, and about others.

About God: He truly will never leave me or forsake me. He is utterly and completely faithful and dependable.

About others: we don't really comprehend how people watch our lives, I think particularly those who claim to follow Jesus, draw attention and inspection especially during crisis. People in this world are desperate for hope. Desperate for truth. Our stories can be used to encourage others in ways we will never know. Also, there are multitudes of individuals who show compassion and reach out during a time of need. I don't take this lightly, and we count ourselves extremely blessed to have so many friends and loved ones who showed us support.

About myself: oftentimes in my life I think I've been characterized as a princess (and not the flattering meaning of the word.). Too often I have escaped hard work and have perhaps appeared as though I had more than my share of blessings. But through this process I learned that when the rubber hits the road, when the toothpaste tube is squeezed, true character comes out. What my parents and God poured into me over the years came out. I'm stronger than I think.

For many many years, my worst fear in life was losing Brian to death. Now I know that regardless of what happens in this lifetime, my

Jesus truly does hold me firm. He will never let go. Therefore, despite the moments when I don't think I can continue to draw breath, I will breathe. Because He is the very breath of life. He, not Brian, is my Life, my Sustainer, my Provider, my Hope.

HOW AM I MORE LIKE JESUS FROM THIS EXPERIENCE?

Wow. I'd have to say the main character trait I see He's developed in me is in the area of being a servant. Not a doormat. Not a slave. But in considering others' needs above my own. (That is not something I've historically been good at. No one wants to make a decision about where to go for dinner? Not a problem. I've probably been hoping for a certain outcome since long before the topic was raised. And I have no problem voicing my opinion!) Servanthood was not a badge I was desiring. Except that Jesus desires it for me. Commands it actually.

I fail miserably. Often. Repeatedly. I serve at times looking gracious on the outside but seething on the inside. Or I serve seething on the outside and whining on the inside. Or at times I actually find that I am serving in joy. Must be His joy. Wow. Okay. Thank you, Jesus.

How could I actually even consider saying that I *don't* regret the stroke? Because my husband has become an even more amazing man. And who he is spiritually today would not have existed without that subarachnoid hematoma which occurred July 10, 2014. The journey we have walked has shaped us and allowed us to minister to others (2 Corinthians 1:3–4). There are **so** many experiences, people, insights, impressions, miracles, blessings, friendships, revelations we would have missed if this pathway had not been presented to us. (Reminds me of the "Welcome to Holland" essay by Emily Kingsley 1987, given to me shortly after Garrett's birth and diagnosis of Down's syndrome.)

I had an interesting experience at the vet yesterday. It was clear that there was a story with the people checking out in front of me. I couldn't tell whether it was husband and wife, woman and father, or perhaps she was a caregiver of some sort. The man looked perhaps senile or that he might have Alzheimer's. They moved back and I was standing facing the counter paying my bill. I then felt very gentle hands on my shoulders and heard the man murmur something. The woman immediately spoke up and moved him away from me apologetically. I casually and cheerfully dismissed it. In the parking lot, she came up to me and said, "My husband has dementia and gets confused. I am so so sorry." The look on her face broke my heart. She was completely washed out, looked utterly exhausted and alone. I said, "It's really okay. My son has special needs and my husband had a stroke three years ago. It didn't bother me at all." Yes, I can now relate to someone in a caregiver role.

There have been hours of emotional pain, free-falling somersaults during which I felt like my heart was on fire ready to explode... or implode. However, because I was able to face the grief, feel the pain, and navigate the pain with the Lord, I've been able to enter into others' grieving to offer an ear, a hug, or a prayer. This I see as an amazing gift gained. Life isn't fair, and it's not easy. Even as Christians, we are not promised a life without pain. (John 16:33). But we are promised an abundant life because Jesus overcame the world. That means he overcame weakness. And death. And pain. And grief. And strokes.

SHEILA'S ACKNOWLEDGEMENTS
SECTION ...

In a journey like this, it is impossible to name everybody who had an impact or who was a blessing to us. We were surrounded by an incredible support system of loving family, friends, neighbors, and church. As has been shared, we were the recipients of so much generosity in many different forms. Sometimes it was people that we knew; oftentimes the source was unknown or anonymous. Please know that we are grateful, and that God used you.

To our sons, Colton and Garrett: we are so proud of the young men you have become! Colton, you took a large stride into manhood and took on responsibility when Dad couldn't. Yet you kept your calm demeanor and quiet trust in the Lord to work everything out. I remember a friend telling me of a conversation she had with you during the first few months of recovery. You told her that you weren't worried about this situation because we weren't worried. That was a huge encouragement and admonition to me, as well as a welcomed confirmation of your personal faith in the Lord. I'm so proud of you, Son, and love you tremendously. Garrett, you remained peaceful, calm, and found joy in any situation most of the time. Your purity and innocence is always inspiring to me. The veil between our physical world and the spiritual realm with Jesus is thinner with you I believe. Because of that you are often such an example of

It's Ok! I Had A Stroke

resting in the moment and taking what comes with quiet but steadfast faith. We love you, buddy, and are so thankful you're our son.

I especially want to thank Claire Hetrick for her excellent editing advice and gracious willingness to allow me to reprint any notes I gleaned from her teachings. A few friends and my dear mother gave initial feedback with rough drafts— it was very helpful to me. Thank you! And to my high school English Teachers, Mrs. Whetzel and Mrs. Stolpe, I'm now very grateful for the stacks of grammar worksheets and volumes of writing that was required!

BRIAN'S ACKNOWLEDGEMENTS SECTION

Through this whole process of writing this book, I was reminded how many people God brought into our lives, both before and after the stroke. Good friends who were with us through the stroke and continue to be with us in prayer, helping us in whatever way we needed, meeting a need when they saw them without being asked most of the time. I can't say enough about our dear friends Bryan and Aimee Patrick. There is no way ever that we could have made it through without those two people. They are two of the greatest and closest friends that I think I've ever had. I know that we will be friends with them for life, no doubt. I love them like they were my own family, and often we have been even closer than blood family. Through this experience, I have seen my relationship with my own brother grown closer, and I've seen him and his wife grow in their relationship with the Lord. What a blessing that has been! Of course my parents have been incredibly supportive, financially when we needed it, rides to therapy and doctor appointments to free Sheila up at times, and basically we knew we could have depended on them in whatever way we needed to. I love them very much and am so grateful! Most of all, I can't thank God enough for my wife. I know now, after twenty-six years, why He had me marry her. She is uniquely equipped to handle the things God throws at her. Together we are better than we are separately. I hope I have many more years with her.

I want to thank all the different physical and occupational therapists I had in the rehab center and later in the outpatient rehab—Amy Gray, Melanie, Kevin, Eva, Eric, Tracy, just to name a few. Oh, and I remember the young speech therapist who had recently graduated. She was a sweetheart. I think I blew her away sometimes. There were so many! I know there's no way I can name everyone.

Our church family did so much for us as well! Friends from all over helped us in many various ways. Chuck and Patricia Berger, Jerry Wilson (who graduated to receive his eternal reward December 2017), Robbie Allison, Michelle Howard, Karel Dill, Bennett Brashier, Marvin Romero, Jayne Guilford, again, just to name a few! There were many people who brought us meals, sent cash or gift cards, groceries, or helped with yardwork. The list is long! Please know that we remember and are so grateful! The Craun family stepped in and had Garrett for hours those first couple months. Somehow my boys were fed and loved on while Sheila ran back and forth. Even as recently as going home for Christmas in 2016, our dear friend Robby Meadows gave me an acoustic bass guitar! Just on the spur of the moment while we were at his recording studio so Sheila could work on a new album, he handed it to me to play and practice on to help improve my dexterity in my hand. What blessings!

And it's not as though I was asking people to help or asking for these things. I was just trusting that whatever God wants me to have, He will provide—either a way for me to buy it, or just that people would have it on their heart to supply it. That's how we're supposed to live in community. Now He's put it on our hearts, as we've experienced abundance here in Texas, to give. It's a blessing to be involved in that process at both ends—the receiving and the giving. It's a blessing to be able to give, and it's a blessing to receive.

Last Page Of The Book

We would love to hear from you! You may contact us via email at shei-lalloydlive2@yahoo.com, or by snail mail at 173 Clubhouse Court, Woodstock, VA 22664 Visit our Facebook page at "IT'S OK I Had a Stroke." Find audio book info on our website at www.sheilalloydlive.com or Amazon. The website has original music as well as devotional writings.

If you or a loved one has suffered a stroke, we would highly recommend contacting Faith Haley, neuro-educational specialist located in Katy, Texas. See www.aBrilliantFoundation.com. (The parent organization is Little Giant Steps, and there are resources all over the country.) We were led to her through one of my young piano students who was in a therapy program with Faith for developmental delays. After a couple phone conversations and then a personal evaluation face to face, we began the program January 2, 2017. It is a program mostly done at home with occasional visits in person. Leaving her office that first day, Brian said, "**This** is why God brought us to Texas!" He has seen amazing improvement already and we look forward to the second half of the program. If the Lord allows, that will be a story for the next book!

Appendix 1

I want to have a relationship with Jesus. How do I start?

First, recognize that you have done wrong things in your life. The Bible calls this sin. We are all sinners, and the Bible says that the penalty for sin is eternal death and separation from God. Romans 3:23 NIV says, *"For all have sinned and fall short of the glory of God."*

But because God loves us he sent Jesus to pay the debt we could never pay. John 3:16 NIV says, *"For God so loved the world that he gave his one and only Son, that whoever believes in him shall not perish but have eternal life."* And Romans 6:23 NIV promises, *"For the wages of sin is death, but the gift of God is eternal life in Christ Jesus our Lord."*

"Salvation" or "being saved" is the term that describes when we believe and accept that Jesus Christ died on the cross to pay for our sins.

There is nothing we can do that would make us good enough for God to forgive us. The wonderful news is that there is nothing we need to do to get salvation; it is a free gift from God! Ephesians 2:8–10 NIV declares, *"For it is by grace you have been saved, through faith —and this is not from yourselves, it is the gift of God— not by works, so that no one can boast. For we are God's handiwork, created in Christ Jesus to do good works, which God prepared in advance for us to do."*

When we accept this gift, God wipes our slate clean and calls us eternally His child. We are never separated from Him again! Romans 8:38–39 NIV paints a dramatic picture of our assurance in Christ: *"For I am convinced that neither death nor life, neither angels nor demons, neither the present nor the future, nor any powers, neither height nor depth, nor anything else in all creation, will be able to separate us from the love of God that is in Christ Jesus our Lord."*

We have the presence of God inside us in the form of the Holy Spirit, and we can have the assurance of eternal life in heaven with God when we die. (John 3:16, and Romans 8:38-39 above. Also, Revelation 21:4 NIV: *"He will wipe every tear from their eyes. There will be no more death or mourning or crying or pain, for the old order of things has passed away."*)

You can pray right now and accept God's gift of salvation! It doesn't matter where you are or what you have done in your life. You do not have to say any magic words; it is not the words that bring salvation, but the belief and the intent of your heart. Here is a suggested prayer you might use, but feel free to modify it and use your own words:

"Dear Jesus, thank you for loving me. I believe that you are God and that you died on the cross for my sins. I believe that you rose from the dead. Please forgive me for everything I've done wrong. I want you to come into my life. Help me to learn more about you. In Jesus' name, amen."

If you prayed this prayer, realize that all of the angels in heaven are rejoicing and over you right now! We would love to hear from you! Please contact us so we can pray for you. Also, if you have made a decision to let Jesus be the Lord of your life, please share that decision with your spiritual director, pastor, priest, or a trusted Christian friend. It is very important that you begin to spend time reading the Bible and being around other Christians in order to grow in this new relationship!

Appendix 2

REFLECTION ON IDENTITY

WHO AM I?

My identity is not in things or what I do.
Neither beauty, fame, nor fortune set my value.
The core of who I am and what I'm worth
Rests with He who formed me before birth.
Your word, Lord, tells plainly who I am in You.
May these truths reshape what I believe is true:

I am blessed, I am chosen,
Forgiven, loved, emboldened.
I am cherished, held, protected, guarded,
Redeemed, treasured, and aptly armored.

Under Your wings is refuge from the storm.
I am safe and can sing when all goes wrong.
I'm equipped for whatever You place before me—
Works You planned before I came to be.
I am guided, molded, transformed,
Filled with Your light—

A shining star in blackest night.
I am gifted as You see fit to give,
Talents to serve You as I live.
Never abandoned or forgotten, I am always on Your mind.
Never walk life's path alone; You promise to lead the blind.
I am holy, even righteous, yes it's true.
My Lord Jesus, all because of You.
I am not bound by time and space.
I'm eternal by Your loving grace.
So when my time on earth is done,
I will worship at Your glorious throne.
Until that day, Lord, let me be
Who You say I am to be.
Remembering Your love for me
Walking in Your identity.

Sheila L. Lloyd, July 2017

Scriptures to study behind this poem:

Jeremiah 1:5;
Psalm 139; Psalm 46
Ephesians 1:3–14; 2:8–10; 6:10–20
2Timothy 1:7;
Zephaniah 3:17;
1John 1:9; 3:1
Isaiah 40:29–31; 41:10,13; 42:6,16; 43:1–3; 43:25; 49:15–16;
Daniel 12:3;
2Corinthians 3:12–18; 4:1–7;
Philippians 2:12–16;
Hebrews 10:19; 13:5

APPENDIX 3

WELCOME TO HOLLAND

by
Emily Perl Kingsley

I am often asked to describe the experience of raising a child with a disability—to try to help people who have not shared that unique experience to understand it, to imagine how it would feel. It's like this...

When you're going to have a baby, it's like planning a fabulous vacation trip—to Italy. You buy a bunch of guide books and make your wonderful plans. The Coliseum. The Michelangelo. David. The gondolas in Venice. You may learn some handy phrases in Italian. It's all very exciting.

After months of eager anticipation, the day finally arrives. You pack your bags and off you go. Several hours later, the plane lands. The flight attendant comes in and says, "Welcome to Holland."

"Holland?!?" you say. "What do you mean Holland?? I signed up for Italy! I'm supposed to be in Italy. All my life I've dreamed of going to Italy."

But there's been a change in the flight plan. They've landed in Holland and there you must stay.

The important thing is that they haven't taken you to a horrible, disgusting, filthy place, full of pestilence, famine, and disease. It's just a different place.

So you must go out and buy new guide books. And you must learn a whole new language. And you will meet a whole new group of people you would never have met.

It's just a different place. It's slower-paced than Italy, less flashy than Italy. But after you've been there for a while and you catch your breath, you look around... and you begin to notice that Holland has wind-mills.....and Holland has tulips. Holland even has Rembrandts.

But everyone you know is busy coming and going from Italy... and they're all bragging about what a wonderful time they had there. And for the rest of your life you will say "Yes, that's where I was supposed to go. That's what I had planned."

And the pain of that will never, ever, ever, ever go away... because the loss of that dream is a very very significant loss.

But... if you spend your life mourning the fact that you didn't get to Italy, you may never be free to enjoy the very special, the very lovely things ... about Holland.